CALISTHENICS

How to Make Your Dream Body and Proven Guide to Get Muscles Create the Physique You Want

(Calisthenics to Look and Feel Your Best From the Boardroom to the Bedroom)

Harry Willian

Published By Jackson Denver

Harry Williams

All Rights Reserved

Calisthenics: How to Make Your Dream Body and Proven Guide to Get Muscles Create the Physique You Want (Calisthenics to Look and Feel Your Best From the Boardroom to the Bedroom)

ISBN 978-1-77485-365-8

Legal & Disclaimer

The information contained in this book is not designed to replace or take the place of any form of medicine or professional medical advice. The information in this book has been provided for educational and entertainment purposes only.

The information contained in this book has been compiled from sources deemed reliable, and it is accurate to the best of the Author's knowledge; however, the Author cannot guarantee its accuracy and validity and cannot be held liable for any errors or omissions. Changes are periodically made to this book. You must consult your doctor or get professional medical advice before using any of the suggested remedies, techniques, or information in this book.

TABLE OF CONTENTS

Introduction

This book outlines the most effective steps and strategies for how to develop and train strength, flexibility, and mobility by doing calisthenics. You don't need use of any equipment.

Calisthenics is a practice that has existed since Ancient Greece and has been utilized to build near-superhuman strength as well as agility and flexibility over the course of time. This book you'll learn some fundamental and intermediate details about the fundamentals behind calisthenics and also the benefits provided by this type of exercise. The book also comes with step-by step instructions to exercises that will build the upper body, core and lower back strength as well as mobility.

This book will guide you through basic routines and more challenging exercises, and along with directions that are simple to follow.

Chapter 1: Why Calisthenics is Important: The Benefits

1-Loss of weight while shaping:

There are many who affirm exercising aerobically is the most efficient method of losing weight. However, they're typically paired with weight-lifting exercises in order to build muscles. Increasing the heart rate and general demands of the body can reduce fat, but it also produces the substance called "glycogen" that is a type of muscle fat. In the process of burning the muscle fat, we lose the bulk of the muscle , but not stimulating it sufficiently to trigger the muscle to increase mass. Therefore, adding weights and resistance training are essential to keep your muscles toned. This can increase the total amount of time required train in the gym to get similar results to those obtained through Calisthenics with shorter amount of time. Calisthenics incorporates aerobic exercise and weight lifting. This makes it the ideal method of losing weight, without sacrificing muscle mass , and also shed weight while gaining weight simply by changing the amount of repetitions you do and the type of exercises you decide to perform.

2. Easier on the mix:

Weight lifting and cardiovascular exercises like uphill running , which is believed to decrease the most amount of weight, are linked to the highest number of joint injuries particularly large joints that are dependent such as elbows and knees joints. Weight lifting makes use of joints as pivots, so any additional weights increase the stress upon the fulcrum (that is the joint) instead of the muscle on its own. Calisthenics, however, provides an equal distribution of weight and the muscle and joints. The use of your own muscles lets your body have an natural progression in the amount of weight to lift. As you gain fitness levels, and with a greater increase in the size of your muscles, you will be able to perform more intense exercises without having to use additional weights which will place a greater strain on your muscles, which could result in bursitis, tendon tears or arthritis.

(Joint inflammation conditions)

3- Increase strength for weightlifters who are beginners:

Before jumping into the iron pumping lifestyle Calisthenics is an essential exercise to build the body's endurance for future lifting, specifically for those who are new to the sport. Calisthenics will ensure that the novice does not overstress their body excessively through a ferocious effort to begin strong. You'll be shocked to learn that lifting weights can bulk your biceps, it does not guarantee that you'll be able to perform pushups or pull-ups like a lean gymnast who has concentrated more on effective muscular contraction, rather than effective muscular endurance to load. Engaging all muscles in an limb is a more effective method to build strength than focusing on training from the beginning because it does not improve the muscles that are smaller and less developed within the body to assist in stabilizing joints. This can lead to the risk of joint pain, especially for beginners.

4- Cost effective

Fitness instructors and gyms are in greater demand than ever before due to the way the media depicts the need to achieve a perfect body and the ease of access to all the junk food, which leads to obesity. This is a perfect base for a profitable business I'm sure you're thinking of it. That's what fitness training has become being: a way of allowing someone else earn money from the need to maintain your health. Calisthenics however costs practically nothing. It requires only a small amount of equipment required for this kind of exercise. The equipment used can be replaced easily making Calisthenics one of the most efficient exercises that can be done at anywhere and at any time you want, while achieving the same results as everybody else in the gym.

It is also possible to perform in a small space, meaning you could get a good exercise right in the park or within the privacy of your own bedroom to make your workout more private. Some people feel that their gym to be a bit stale with their peers even though they may be being more successful than they are which can cause a decline in motivation to exercise, especially when results take time to appear. It is possible to do Calisthenics on vacation , so you don't need to be concerned about returning with an unsatisfied stomach to tackle. In actual Calisthenics is among only a handful of exercises that do not cause muscle flaccidity once it ceases this is the second advantage of this amazing way of exercising.

5- Strengthening without the fear of losing strength once exercising has been stopped This is a frequent issue for weightlifters. you must constantly lift in order to keep the muscle structure you have created. The appealing muscle build-up after weight lifting is actually your body's way of compensating with the stress of. The sudden increase in weight on muscles results in stretching of the fibers in the muscle to a point beyond the strain imposed on muscles causes them to adapt to increase their size and reducing their energy expenditure in order to withstand the strain. If you stop this type of exercise, it causes muscles to keep metabolizing in a lower level of energy and not making use of the extra weight that is gained. This causes the phenomenon known as "disuse atrophy" of muscles that are isolated, which can makes the muscle you gained weak and stiff after you've stopped this type of exercise. Calisthenics, however, does not cause stretching of muscle fibers since it is an evenly distributed weight distribution across the limbs. Therefore, it utilizes the method of exercise that includes "isometric" contraction, which keeps myofibrils of identical in length but encourages them to make use of more energy to sustain the contraction through the burning of more calories. It also decreases the chance of muscle sagging when the stimuli of excessive burden has been removed.

6- Training the mind and body

Calisthenics is not just about building strength , but also stimulates the mind to improve coordination and orientation which improves mental health and improves your ability to think. By challenging your body with more exercises that are not monotonous, repetitive will stimulate not only your brain's motor cortex , but also the higher functional regions of the brain which assist you to keep your balance and allow your ability to find more efficient ways to support your weight and maintain the position for longer. This boosts your mental wellbeing as well as your awareness, which causes you to be more prepared to handle difficult situations, by creating an ideal state of mind. It challenges you to the limits and gives you a sense of satisfaction. There is nothing more satisfying than knowing your body and understanding how it's the most effective tool you can rely on.

7- Variation:

It also offers variety so that you won't be doing the same boring routines again and repeatedly. Actually, the fact that it is used as a group exercise can make it more enjoyable and helps you to improve in other sports of the team too.

8-Speed: So what happens if you lift the weight of your brother?

Have you noticed that your average muscled person is in reality a slow walker, and won't be the front of the pack to be first in the marathon? It's because the development of muscles like the ones of bodybuilders adds to weight and requires an extra effort to perform more rapid movements at joints since there is more pressure. Calisthenics can limit the extent that you can increase muscle mass. And since it's combined with gross motor exercises which also incorporate a range of agility and flexibility exercises, it doesn't limit the speed you can move. In fact , the aerobic aspect of Calisthenics will ensure that you keep the right level of agility throughout your exercise.

Chapter 2: Setting Your Fitness S.M.A.R.T. Goals.

"A goal that is properly established is half-way reached." Zig Ziglar. Zig Ziglar

If you wish to succeed in everything you do, it is essential set goals. Goals are what motivate people and allows them to feel motivated to do something, however when people set their resolutions for the New Year of losing weight , they typically set their goals in a vague manner. The goal is to shed weight, look great for summer, look slim or slim, etc... I will clarify that if you are one of them and you haven't reached your fitness goals yet it is not your fault.

When you are trying to establish goals, there is a specific method for the process. This technique is known as "S.M.A.R.T. goal setting". The name implies it's a more deliberate method for creating your fitness goals. Once you've learned this technique, you'll never return to the old method of setting goals and will finally achieve your New Year's resolution.

S.M.A.R.T goal setting must include the following details.

S - Specific: You need to know exactly what you are trying to achieve. (Example I'm trying to shed 10lbs I'd like to perform the muscle up, I'd like for all 6 parts of my abs in front of me etc. ...)

M - Measurable The goal should be quantifiable, preferably with a numerical value. (Example, weight, reps, sets, etc...)

A Attainable: You have to believe that you will attain your goal.

realistic: The objective should be achievable enough that you are able to see yourself reaching the goals you've established for yourself.

The Timeline: define a precise timeframe for your target (Example that you want to achieve it by the close in the calendar year)

After following the guidelines in the S.M.A.R.T acronym, you will be able to achieve an objective such as:

I'd like to lose 15lbs of pure fat before July 15th without loosing any muscle

I'd like to do 20 pull ups before the end of the year , while getting that V-Taped body I've always longed for.

I'd like to do an entire muscle-up before June 15 to amaze my friend.

These examples all follow the guidelines above for S.M.A.R.T goals. Therefore, before moving into the next chapter, I would like you to come up with your own list of SMART goals you'd like to reach this year. After you've accomplished your SMART goal , move onto the next chapter.

Chapter 3: What is Calisthenics?

To reap the maximum degree from this book it is essential to know the basics of what Calisthenics is as well as what it's not and what it could offer to you, and what it isn't able to offer you in the present. Before we get into the specifics we'll take a quick stroll through the history of Calisthenics.

Calisthenics originates from the Greek term "kallos," which means beauty in addition to "sthenos," which means power. When you combine these two words together, it could be described as creating art with just your body weight, inertia and gravity to improve your physical form.

The origins of Calisthenics go back to the beginning of evolution of humans, when humans were required to run, walk and jump, lunge or roll and pull to survive. Modern equipment for gyms has been designed on these methods of survival to work the muscle groups that surround your body. This is the reason Calisthenics is generally regarded as "the most natural and easy form of workout" for your body to do. Even homo sapiens' cousins such as the monkey or apes, do this type of exercise to strengthen their chest, arm and back muscles.

At the time of the ancients, Calisthenics was also used as the primary source of physical fitness for armies, militias and soldiers. It was the most efficient method to train soldiers and teach them to collect, organize and work in a team. There was always something spiritual and not just in terms of being conscious of your body but also in sharing that kind of connection with others.

The bodyweight exercise that is slow and targeted muscle activation and improved flexibility in time, led to the most famous master of fitness currently that is the gymnast. In addition to lifting weights and running long distances, many gymnasts train for up to 30 hours every week, using only their own body weight, inertia and a purposeful, deliberate movement.

With the advancement of technological advancements and the spread of gymnastics competitions across the globe in addition to the Olympics the sport of exercise has been gaining popularity. The stars of social media have been offering more information about their exercise routines, shining the light on Calisthenics and the benefits this type of exercise is for the body. Furthermore, Calisthenics are the easiest exercise "forms" for athletes to record and post on social media as they don't require gym equipment, gym memberships or classes. Anyone can perform it at home, and keep up by sharing their workout videos.

Wikipedia offers the following definition for calisthenics:

"Calisthenics is an exercise that consists of a variety of gross motor activities that include pushing, standing or running. They are typically done in a rhythmic manner and using minimal equipment, such as as an exercise that is based on body weight. They aim to improve strength and fitness as well as flexibility by the use of jumping, pulling, squatting or swinging and any other activity that utilizes your body's natural weight. Calisthenics could bring the benefits of aerobic and muscular conditioning as well as improving psychomotor abilities like agility, balance and coordination."

At its heart, Calisthenics is the most naturaland pure type of exercise. It's something people have been practicing for hundreds of years. It's not about expensive apparatus, memberships to gyms or classes that are specialized. It's about getting an individual's body, and moving in carefully planned jumps, bursts of energy, running, or squats, to work various muscle groups to improve fitness as well as reduction in weight, improved agility and so on.

Since Calisthenics is innate to us as a fitness technique, teams of athletes as well as military units, Olympians and professional athletes are also involved in some form of Calisthenics in their training. Teams in particular join as a team to increase connection and discipline. This is similar to what you might have done during your fitness classes as a kid.

Example: Lu Xiaojun. Lu Xiaojun can grab up 176kg, clean and jerk up to 204kg, and he attributes all his achievements to the Calisthenics. The Olympian stated that slow, deliberate bodyweight building and bodyweight involvement the base of his power and his current success and not some expensive gym equipment.

What is the reason for Calisthenics?

Calisthenics is, in every aspect considered to be a "low effort" type of exercise. In the COVID-19 world, we all require things that are low-fuss as well as low-stress and accessible. So, many more than are searching for these types of workouts on social media. It's the principal method for working out.

However, beyond coronavirus and the current scenario that we are in and the current situation, we'd like to discuss the advantages and disadvantages of this kind of exercise engagement to ensure that you are fully aware of what you can be expecting. Let's begin with the benefits.

The Benefits of Calisthenics:

Everyone can do Calisthenics Every person in the world regardless of how naturally skilled and fit or tough they may be they can perform Calisthenics. Everyone has been trained to do an exercise with body weight regardless of whether they are taking a walk up the stairs or getting your body up from the bed. If you're elderly or disabled, or is overweight, they may still take part in exercise that's appropriate the body. The intensity can be customized to suit the individual and the duration of an exercise. If one person is able to perform ten jump in a row it's still Calisthenics. If someone else is able to perform 500 jump jacks at once and still be able to do 500, it's still Calisthenics. Even if you're not able to do the actual push-up, however then you can stand on the ground with your knees bent and do a different version that involves the body through bodyweight exercises. Isn't that amazing?

It's more secure than gym Equipment Do you look at the dangers of gym equipment? If one cables snapped or structures made of metal broken, individuals could be killed. In Calisthenics it's more difficult to hurt yourself. First of all there's no fancy fitness equipment is around now. Furthermore, you are able to only perform what your body is able to handle at the moment So, when you attempt to do push-ups upside down but you're not able to have the strength to do it the body will collapse. Additionally, if you add the barbell to your exercise, you have the possibility of straining or pulling your muscles. In other words, you extend beyond your body's capacity to support itself. In Calisthenics you can only do what you can do in the time frame you are given. It's the most secure method of exercising, particularly for those who are unfamiliar with the world of fitness.

Exercises can be scaled up The majority of people think that equipment for gyms is the best method to increase the weight and increase muscles. It's simple - you simply add weight. But what people aren't aware of is that the same principle is applicable to exercises using body weight.

Modifications can be made to enhance the difficulty of an exercise. In addition, the slower you move such as a push-up the more difficult it will be. By focusing on quantity over quality the Calisthenics program can put muscles in the same manner of push-back with weights as fitness equipment. However, with Calisthenics you're paying attention to your body and what it is able to do and reducing the risk of injuries.

Multi-faceted Strength Results: Calisthenics gives your body far more than muscles that are strong You can apply those new techniques and brain-body connections to other activities, sports such as hiking, trips and more. The majority of calisthenics exercises instruct the body to be in sync. This helps ensure that there's an interaction between all parts of your body, enhancing coordination, awareness, as well as flexibility. The skills you learn are applicable to other activities, sports such as traveling, travel and other activities. You may even become more alert If you've lived your entire life in the cloud.

Unique Strength Targeting We're all aware about triceps, biceps quads, and hamstrings but few people know about the smaller, less important muscles that make up a part of the muscle-skeletal system. By doing Calisthenics you're using a lot of isometric workouts that target specific muscle groups while using other muscles. When you do an isometric workout, you can pull the door into place for a minute. Instead of being concerned about how many repetitions you're getting the first place, you're in this one position in order to engage all the muscles that are engaged in a precise manner. There are more muscles engaged in these exercises too, which helps those who belong to specific groups connect and align more smoothly.

The drawbacks of Calisthenics:

It isn't possible to be perfect in this world. That's the reason we need to be honest about any possible problems that may arise in Calisthenics.

Low Body Muscle Growth Massive Issues In terms of weight, it's difficult to develop enormous quads, hamstrings and quads with no external help. This is due to the fact that your lower body is designed to support your body's weight so engaging it using your own weight may not yield significant muscle gains. Single-leg squats, bodyweight lunges, squats as well as hamstring curls, are all great exercises for keeping your lower body lean and more toned. However, if you wish to see your muscles burst through your pants then you're going to require a amount of weight, or even two.

Weights are not able to be added to increase resistance The purpose for Calisthenics is to exercise without the heavy 100-pound weights you'll find on bars. Thus, in Calisthenics you must be an extra creative approach to your workouts to increase the intensity. This is what keeps people from trying it at all It can appear as if it's too hard. In the current COVID-19 world, lots of people have no alternative this is the reason they're willing to study.

Critics claim that That a Big Muscle Mass isn't possible While this is disputated, it's beneficial to discuss it with you There are some who argue that huge muscle gains are not achievable using bodyweight alone. Numerous athletes have debunked this idea and shown that, with patience and time the body can certainly increase muscle mass. If you're looking for an incredible, superhuman strength, then you're likely to have to lift some weights. Be aware that if you exceed the capacity of your body, you're at risk of injury.

Why Calisthenics Are Unique

Once we've got completed our work, let's close this section by looking at some of the ways that the exercise routine will benefit your body specifically. There are many amazing advantages that result from giving up the machines and saying hello to your body's natural shape. Here are a few that you should consider:

Get your hands out when it comes to Calisthenics hand is involved in virtually every movement and motion. Hands are utilized to push, pull and even participate in core workouts, which means that your sensitivity in your wrists and hands will increase. Through body-building and other forms of exercise, you just connect the equipment onto your wrist and let your body to take over the rest. However, with Calisthenics you'll be focused on your hands constantly which will improve your the strength of your hand and improve the overall brain-body connection of your body.

Core Engagement The core is an essential part that makes up your entire body. When you are using the latest equipment at the gym, their metal structures can shift the majority on top your body, which could leave your core sleeping. The core of your body is connected to your body, and serves as a the majority of your power and strength. When you practice Calisthenics because the majority exercises require stability and balance your core will be active in each exercise. Your core plays crucial roles in the development and growth that you can achieve strength.

Scapula Engagement among all the regions of your body performing callisthenic activities the scapula is one important factor to consider. The key to strength in your upper body doesn't originate from shoulder or chest muscles. It actually is in your back. The scapula of your back is connected to your clavicle and provides an anchor bone for your body to support the rib cage. It offers stability for your upper extremities, along with the ability to elevate, depress, upward or downward movement, as well as protraction and retraction of your body.The scapula also serves as an important point of attachment for the ball-and-socket joint within your shoulder. In essence using your scapula to engage it and working the back muscles could give you more benefits than you think.

Straight Arm Strength particular strength, exactly as it sounds, happens when there is strength in the elbow that is locked. This puts a tremendous tension on the arm as well as its connective tissues like the biceps and bicep tendon. It's an excellent method to build up arm muscles without lifting or roll any weights. Straight arm pulls strengthens the back.

Calisthenics is a form of exercise that is the practice of training the nervous system along and with muscles. It is likely that you will not be able to simply continue to do exercise without contemplating the exercises and the body position. Controlling this type of exercise over your body can strengthen your connection to the nervous system , and the functions it performs within your body.

Once we've laid the groundwork regarding Calisthenics, the benefits and why you should be concerned about it, you should know more about nutrition and how your diet choices can have direct effects on your fitness performance.

Chapter 4: Beginner Tier One

Month One

The following workout routines are a mix and match according to which one you enjoy the best. Focus your efforts to target the main muscle groups during each workout. This includes abs, arms, legs and chest, as well as back. By focusing on each part of your body, each exercise session is a sure way to get full body results. Once you begin making a goal of working out at least three times each week.

It is not realistic to expect huge outcomes after one months (or more or less) of exercise. Take a look at the time it took you to get to where you are today, and then give your body a little slack and you'll see the improvements sooner than you believe. When performing each of the exercises listed below, it is crucial to take less time resting between exercises as is possible to get the most benefit. This month is going to set the stage for coming months. Make it count.

New Exercises

Chinupsor Close-grip chinups This exercise is done in similar to the pullup, however when you reach out for the bar, you use your fingers facing towards you instead of away towards your. Lean back on the bar and then get your elbows lower while maintaining your arms in the closest position to each other as you can. Chinups that are regular should be done by laying your hands at shoulder width, and close-grip chinups are done with hands that are almost touching.

Wall sit: Start by placing your back approximately 2 feet away from the wall, then leaning forward and lowering yourself until your and the wall are as close to an angle of 90 degrees as is possible. You should have your feet spread out at an arm's length, with your feet equally distributed.

Chair dip Begin by sitting at the edge of the chair, stretching your feet out towards the front so that they touch. Put a hand on the opposite one of your chairs. raise yourself up off the chair before lowering yourself to the floor. Stop when your elbows are 90 degrees.

Inclinate/Decline pushups are the same as regular pushups . However, when you do decline pushups, you put something under your feet to ensure they're elevated. With the incline pushups, you raise your arms.Plank as you would in a normal pushup posture, but rest your forearms and keep your elbows bent in front of you. Relax those muscles that are in the middle. Lunges: Begin by standing and then stepping forward with one leg , making an exaggerated movement until your front foot forms an angle of 90 degrees. Make sure to keep your back straight, and work the core muscles.

Mountain climbers: Begin by placing your body into a position of pushups before pulling the other leg to the side like you're running a race. The workout is done by quickly switching which leg is being pulled forward by moving it between back and back.

Pike Pushups: Begin the exercise by adopting a traditional pushup posture, and then moving your hands towards the ground until you are at a sharp 90 degree angle. Lean toward the side until you're level with your hands. Lower your body until your head nearly gets to the ground.

Australian pulling ups: This workout is similar to a standard pullup, however it is done with the bar being several feet away from the ground. You can grip the bar in the same way as you would normally before putting your feet toward the ceiling and then using both arms and your body to push your chest toward the bar.

Full body workout

The list should be run 3 times in succession, taking up to 4 minutes to rest between exercises. It is okay to allow yourself as long as 1 minute between each exercise , but don't take longer than what you'll need to get forward as your goal is to complete the list as fast as you can.

Begin by doing 3 chinups.

Do a wall sit for 30 seconds

Do 12 dips with the chair

Do 8 squats

Do 8 pushups.

Do 2 pull-ups

Perform 3 leg raises

Perform 7 decline pushups

No equipment for full body workout

Complete the list four times in a row ,
taking up to three minutes to rest
between sets. You are free to take up to
45 seconds of relax between each
workout, but don't take longer than you'll
need to finish the task because the goal is
to complete the list as fast as you can.

Begin by holding the plank for as long as is
possible.

Do 8 squats

Perform 8 lunges

Do 8 pushups.

Perform 8 leg raises

Do as numerous mountain as is possible

Do 8 pushups with pike.

A full body routine that is extra-strength

The list should be run 6 at a time taking up
to two minutes to rest between exercises.
You are free to take as long as 30 seconds

of rest between each workout, however, do not spend longer than you'll have to do because the goal is to complete the list as fast as you can.

Begin by performing 15 pushups on incline.

Do a plank for as long as is possible

Perform jumping jacks every one minute

Do 6 dips

Do 15 Squats

Perform 10 Australian pullups

Perform six chinups that are close-grip.

Month Two

The following workout routines can be combined and matched according to which one you enjoy most. Focus your efforts to work the major muscle areas in every workout, including legs, abs, arms and back, and chest. Concentrating on each part of your body, each workout, will guarantee you will see full body improvements. This month, you are able to mix and mix and match any month-one routines with the following routines. Do your best to do at least three times each week. You can also make one of the days a double, where you can combine either the complete workout routine, or the routine that does not require equipment with another workout that you like.

New exercises

100-meter run: Here are a few points to keep in mind to ensure you're running in a proper manner. The first thing to remember is not to stretch your stride further than you would normally, so concentrate on walking lightly and taking small strides. A good posture is equally important and so is keeping your arm in a controlled position. It is also important to stay clear of putting too much stress in the muscles, and to stay away from landing excessively on your heels or your toes.

Alternating high knees: Begin in a standing position with feet about shoulder-length and with your hands in front of you , as like they are resting on a counter. Then, quickly lift one knee until it touches your hands. Then, switch with the opposite knee when your first foot touches the ground.

Wide/close pushups Pushups are similar to traditional pushups, but instead of having your hands placed at the shoulder width, you can either put your hands at the double shoulder distance for wider pushups, or make sure your elbows are kept tucked to do close pushups.

Upper body workout
The list should be run through 3 times in succession, giving yourself up to four minutes of rest between each attempt. Take as little time between each workout as you can.
Begin by performing 10 pushups.
Do 6 Chinups
Perform 3 chair dips
Do 6 pull-ups
Make 6 dips
Fat burning routine
The list should be run through 4 times in a row , giving yourself up to two minutes to rest between sets. It is okay to allow yourself as long as 30 seconds of rest between each workout, but don't take longer than what you'll need to get

forward as your goal is to complete the list as fast as you can.

Begin with 100 meters of running

Make 5 dips

Do jumping Jacks for 45 seconds

Do 8 pushups.

Alternate high knees and knees for 30 seconds.

Do climbing mountaineers for 30 seconds

Plank for 15 seconds for 15 seconds.

Chest routine

Complete the list four times in a row , giving yourself up to 3 minutes to rest between sets. You are free to take as long as 30 seconds of rest between each workout, but don't take longer than what you'll need to get ahead, as the aim is to complete the list as fast as you can.

Do 10 pushups wide

Do 10 pushups close to each other.

Perform 8 decline pushups

Do 10 pushups a day.

Do 5 dips

Perform 15 pushups with an incline.

Plank for 15 seconds for 15 seconds.

Chapter 5: Calisthenics as advertised

After you have established a solid foundation by doing the fundamental and intermediate calisthenics exercises in earlier chapters, it's time to move on to the details of the calisthenics community. We have all heard of Calisthenics as athletes who can do amazing feats, like the olympic gymnastic athletes who spin and twirl across the air. But, Calisthenics is in essence total control of your body through the use of stabilizing muscles in the core. The next chapter will focus on the core stabilizer muscles. we'll continue to study how to progress through the various methods : muscle-up front lever, muscle-up, and planche.

In my last post, I talked about getting involved with this Calisthenic community. This is due to the fact that the advancements in these exercises, you will need to move out of the comfort of your home most of the time. It is necessary to go to the local park which has a selection of broad-grip pull-up bar and bars that are vertical. In outdoor settings, trying to improve in these calisthenic exercises should not be an issue for you. It is possible to come in contact with people who are with different levels of experience in Calisthenics and those who have made further progress usually will be willing to share their experiences and advice to help you move that more quickly whether it's reworking your technique or boosting your competitive streak.

This time, we will focus on energetic movements (energetic and powerful) first.

Bar Muscle-up

It is a technique which combines a pull up and a dip into a active move. For beginners it is common to use momentum and kipping is commonly employed and has become a common practice , and has earned the name of a typical muscle-up. Professionals who are skilled remove momentum and kipping during this move, and that exercise is referred to as an absolute muscle-up. In this book , we'll discuss the process for regular muscles-up. Begin by hanging over a bar in the overhand position, similar to one of the standard pull-up.

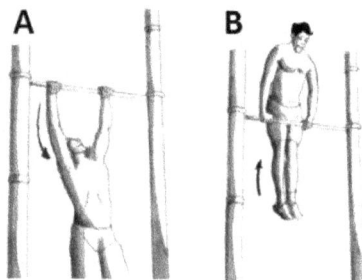

Then, with a powerful pull up, you will reach your chest. This section can be assisted by initially swaying your legs and torso towards the bar. Wait until the direction of your body changes forward. When your upper body is advancing toward the bar while not losing your momentum rapidly flex your wrists as well as elbows over the bar to get yourself into the position of a dip in the bottom.

From there, you can move your body 10-20 degrees to the left or right of the bar, and then perform the ascension portion of the dip . You can do this by keeping your arms straight and activating your triceps.

* Lower yourself slowly to prevent injuries.

If you are unable to perform this exercise, I'd recommend you to explore these strategies for progression.

Create a strong foundation by doing:

* strict pull-upskipping pull-up chest-to-bar pull-up

* parallel bar dips single bar dips

Use a box or a chair to exercise.

* Set the chair or the box in a stable place under the bar.

Perform a part movement of the muscle-up, jumping into the exercise. Make sure not to hurt yourself while doing this, since jumping into any exercise can make the exercise more easy to complete, but it also increases the chances of injuries.

Front lever

This lever the essence of a static move (lock as well as hold) however it begins in a pull-up position which is why I'll call it an energetic move. The motion for the front lever is done by keeping the body and the extremities straight and locked, while moving the body in a straight line to the floor. The face of your body towards towards the sky or the ceiling. This is one of the most difficult one and requires a solid core and back strength.

Begin by hanging over a bar using the overhand position similar to the pull-up.

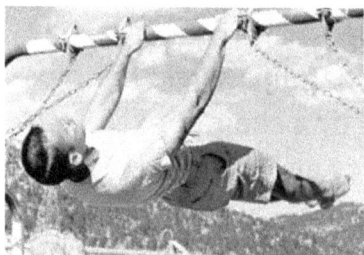

While you do this, bring your knees towards your chest in a way that you are perpendicular with your waist (making an angle of 90 degrees with your thighs and your torso) as you move your body in a straight line to the ground. You can also shift your body backwards to ensure that your hands are more closely to the waist and not your shoulders.

From this point then extend your knees and move your legs to straighten until your body is fully aligned with the floor.
* Keep this position in place by engaging your core. Feel the burning in your abs as well as the gaze of admiration from all people who are watching.

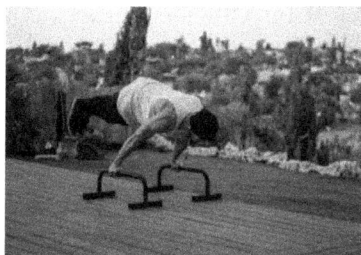

If you're not able to complete the exercise, attempt these techniques for progression. Create a strong foundation by doing:
* leg raiseshanging leg raises dragon flags*
*Dragon flags are like leg raises but you lift the entire mid back until your toes instead of only legs. This exercise is done by lying on a flat floor or bench with something to support your body over your head. Stabilizing your body by gripping the bench to either side of your head.

Engaging your abdominal muscles by raising your legs and hips at 45-60 degrees, then dropping them back down.

* parallel bar dips single bar dips

* Make use of a chair or a box to exercise.

* Set the chair or the box in a secure position beneath the bar.

* Perform a part movement of the muscle-up, jumping into the exercise . Make sure not to hurt yourself by doing this, as jumping into any exercise can make the exercise more easy to do, but also increase the chances of injuries.

* Use stretch bands to help support your legs. (you can find some here: http://amzn.to/2wF5ZP3)

* Loop the band onto the bar and then step into the band, or place it under your ankles or calves.

* Maintain the assisted lever for the longest you can to increase stamina and strength.

Planche

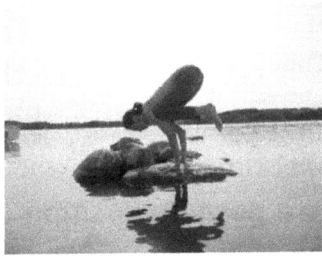

The Planche is a exercises that is static. This exercise puts your body muscles to the test, and primarily engages the abdominal, chest and shoulder muscles. The Planche is achieved by having the body held in a solid position and straight to the ground with legs and back straight . This is a technique that requires balance and stretches all muscles of the body to execute.

There are many different forms of Planche. Due to the physical requirements, it may take a few months or several years, to learn how to use the Planche in its finest shape. It is usually started by studying the frog standing technique in yoga prior to learning the Planche is mastered, so we'll begin with that.

It is important to begin by warming your wrists. This is crucial because they will be submerged to your entire body weight within a short time.

* Move into a push up position.

* Move both feet forward, and bring knees closer the elbows. The knee joint in the middle of each leg on the elbow that is next to it.

Slowly bend your elbows and lift your feet up off the floor. Move your head upwards and then downwards. Be aware not to over-correct and fall on your face or head.

"Balance and Hold.

* As you grow and strengthen your move, you can advance to advanced frog standing by lifting your elbows away from your knees and using your core muscles to raise and balance yourself.

If you're at ease and ready to tackle the Planche this is the order for the move. Start by tucking the Planche. Utilize two parallel bars for this exercise, or you could make use of the tricep dip station that is found in most parks gym space.

* Tucked Planche position Start by lifting yourself to the upright position of dip.

Note: *Tuck knees into your chest, your ankles to your butt, and then lean towards the front. Keep your balance and hold them.

Arms remain straight, locked in. The body is leaning 5-10 degrees forward, which means that shoulders are not directly beneath your hands, but further forward. The back of your body should lie in line with the floor and there should be an incline in your spine due to your legs being bent and snuggled into your torso.

Advanced tucked posture - Once you're at ease with tucked Planche move from the normal tucked Planche position to an advanced Tucked Planche posture by straightening the back to the fullest extent and lowering your knees until they are parallel to the ground , with your thighs and back making an 90 degree angle. Keep and balance

* One Leg Planche From the advanced tuck position just one leg straight to align

with your spine. The other leg remains tucked in to assist in maintaining balance.

* You'll notice that your head moves farther away from the hands. This is normal. If you're unable to keep your weight with this position and you are unable to keep your hands straight you should not extend your legs fully. Move forward once you are able to be able to hold the weight.

* Straddle Planche If you are on one leg Planche It is now time to move to the next leg, but it's simpler if your legs are spread out more.

* Slowly lift the other leg to a bent posture and extend the leg and away from the opposite leg.

Hold and balance.

* Full Planche When you've been able to keep the strapping Planche for more than 30 minutes, you are able to try to reduce the gap between you legs.

Then slowly increase the distance until you've reached the point where your ankles meet.

If you're not able to complete the exercise, Try these strategies for progression.

* Establish a solid foundation by doing:

* planks that have arms fully extended. Core tightplanks that have legs elevated on a seat planks stretch resistance bands tethered to a bar or fixture above your head to help support your legs

You can strengthen your core with a static leg raises. Perform various exercises for your abdominals and oblique that are weighted.

Chapter 6: Most Effective Calisthenic exercises for your back The Suction

If you're like many people, you might have a tendency to ignore your back muscles.

We live in a society that is dominant and are focused on the future that are ahead. In the process, we can create muscle imbalances that are present between the front that we are on and the back.

The positive news is:

The body weight library exercises includes several of the most effective pulling techniques to build muscles in the back and correct imbalances.

We will look at the top ones later on.

We'll begin by...

The Standard Pull-Up

The pull-up is a reference to the upper part of the body, the knee bend is to the lower body.

It is an excellent test in upper back strength. It strengthens the rear into a worn map.

A majority of people do this exercise incorrectly. It is important to concentrate upon getting your body up to the bar, not your chin!

I've seen athletes do all they can to ensure they have their chins over the bar. Keep in mind that we're training our backs and not our necks.

Please don't become one of them.

Exercises for the back of the neck that can be done at a calisthe

A lot of you won't be able to complete just one pull-up.

It's a good thing. Below is a list excellent bodyweight exercises that will aid you in doing your first pull-up.

1.) Wall pulls

Find a wall or a door that is just 8 inches in width so that you are able to easily access both sides.

Be sure to hold it with confidence. Get your feet closely to your wall is possible and hold your arms extended, which forces the weight of your body backwards.

Retract your back to the wall, and then pinch your shoulder blade towards the top. Return slowly to the starting point.

2) Pull-up negatives

This is among my favorites exercises. You should look for a box, or bench which permits you to jump all up to the highest point of the pull-up exercise.

Then slowly (and I'm talking slow) lower yourself to your outstretched arms. At minimum 5 seconds to complete the descent. Repeat.

3) Foot-supported pull-ups

In this instance, search for a chair or a box which you can place behind the bar to take off a portion or all of it. Put your legs down onto the supports and use your heels raise yourself.

Pull-up a negative and lower yourself back to your starting point.

4) Pull-ups

Once you are comfortable with the other variations that are scaled Pull-ups are a great method to master the pull-up.

The exercises are almost the identical. Instead, you employ the grip of an underhand or supination.

They are a bit easier than pull-ups due to the fact that you increase arm strength using the grip of your underhand. If you are able to do pull-ups, you should also be in a position to pull-ups well.

The reversed row or horizontal pull-up

This is a great exercise for those who don't have the pull-up bar.

They can be carried out at a table in the kitchen (just ensure that you have someone or something to support the other end to make sure).

You can improve your difficulty in the vertical chin-up exercise by changing from a version that has a bent knee to one that has straight knees.

Back gymnastics with Calisthenics for advanced students.

You might be among one of the elite 20% of people and could easily do more than 12 times of clean pull-ups that are full of motion.

If yes, find out how to proceed.

Close-Grip Pull-Ups

The more your hands are moving, the harder your arms must do in order to lift the bar.

Move your hands closer and closer until you are able to do pull-ups by keeping your hands touching.

Chest-to-rod pull-ups

This type of variation can increase the level of difficulty since you need to ensure that your chest is physically contact the bar throughout every repetition. It is possible that you will require some extra momentum to assist yourself however, it's important not to go too far.

Like the dynamic push-ups, this workout can aid in training explosive strength.

The pull-up with a wide grip

The pull-ups that have a large handle focus more in the growth of your upper back muscles, particularly that of the lattissimus Dorsi. Set your hands on the side 2 inches more than your shoulder width.

The L-Pull-Up

This exercise is simple. You extend your legs in front of you and create an L-shape using your body. Chin-ups are what you normally do, but keep the L-shape.

This exercise aids in stabilizing your body and stimulate the core muscles.

Advanced back exercises for calisthenics

Then, you'll discover the most advanced gymnastics workouts to strengthen your back.

Pseudo 1-arm pull-ups

You can also define. Take the bar in one hand and place it underneath your palm, and then grasp your forearm using another hand. Create as numerous as you can on each side.

1 Arm Pull-ups with assistance

Place a towel on the bar. Grab the towel using one hand, and your bar using the second hand. The bar's hand must work harder. The farther you lower the towel the more difficult the workout gets.

It is important to make sure to train each side equally.

Weighted pull-ups

If you can master all of these different variations. There is nothing more to do except to add an external resistance. It is possible to do this.

1.) 1 weighted vest

2.) An underwater belt that has chain

3.) One dumbbell placed between legs crossed

Muscles up

Another excellent pull-up variant is the one that uses the muscles upwards. This is a difficult workout, therefore if haven't mastered the other moves don't attempt this.

Do you remember the pull-ups with bar and breasts the past?

To increase muscle mass, you must to be able bring your waist up to the bar!

From this position , you can easily move your elbows up and move to a body weight-lowering position.

Try this out at your home.

Typewriter pull-ups

By using the typewriter pull-up, you get very close to effectiveness of pull-ups with a single arm. Make sure to only try this when you are at ease with pull-up exercises generally.

This is a good thing, it completes the train section.

We can move to the vertical push to create shoulders that are more durable than boulders.

Chapter 7: Key Areas That Should Be Considered for Beginners Calisthenics Exercise

Since Calisthenics is a specific type of exercise and training that has its own advantages and drawbacks, and I'd like to spend some time to review these aspects here. These are due to the manner in which calisthenics exercises utilize the muscles of the body and also the equipment employed, or not being used. This means that it is possible to utilize Calisthenics to enhance the forms of endurance and strength that could not be achieved naturally or through other methods.

Hand Strength

One of the most unique aspects of Calisthenics is the fact that nearly every exercise that we study involves hands. Pulling, pushing, and the core exercises all rely on hands to an extensive extent. Additionally, since Calisthenics emphasizes complete control and strength of the entire body, supporting devices like hooks and belts aren't employed in any way. It is different from the bodybuilding or other types of weighted of exercise which use belts to aid people in staying on pull-up bars, while hooks are employed to keep the barbell in place as it swells up to its limit. It is not difficult to see the practice being carried out in gyms, and by everyone trying to build muscle. Hooks as well as braces is part as a part of game for bodybuilders. They tend to strike other muscles, and they do not want their hands, which means forearms, get tired until the muscle that they use becomes tired. Additionally, we as those who practice Calisthenics require the arms and hands to be as sturdy as is physically possible and in turn and the grip. This is completely logical when you give it a second thought. You might have the most powerful hands in the world however, it's useless in the event that your forearms and hands aren't strong enough to withstand the force and utilize it. I am a firm believer that I am able to rely on my hands that I've created a whole book about the subject. It's known as GRIP.

Hands are used during calisthenics for a variety of tasks such as holding onto the floor and hold your body weight as well as use a pull-up bar to hang on objects, or move from one place to the next with sheer force rather than speed. These activities all depend heavily on the strength and endurance of the the hand as well as finger strength. If you're lacking that strength ability, you're probably not in a position to perform any of the more complex calisthenics exercises. Of of course, there are a variety of exercises for hand and finger strength that could be utilized to target specific muscles involved in gripping, however a lot of the strength required be gained through performing the simple exercises that I've listed in the section on exercises.

THE CORE

The heart is an area of our body that, through time, has experienced many fad equipment and exercises that I believe we can all agree that the majority of them are a waste of time. Contrary to what the majority of people believe as well as what news media will claim, performing hundreds of crunches or sit-ups aren't going to build a strong heart. Sitting ups and crunches aren't going to burn fat off your midsection, either. Regarding what it requires to improve it is the same as every other fiber of muscle. To grow stronger the muscle must contract in response to a force and the resistance needs to increase over time to increase the strength. Note that and remember that it's not the number of repetitions that needs to rise, it's the resistance that has to grow. That means no matter the number of sit-ups that you do in the event that you don't boost that resistance level, you will never grow stronger.

In the traditional way of exercising the core is viewed as an integral area of the body that can improve the appearance. Abs are emphasized and diets are strictly maintained, and everyone wants to get a six-pack. The heart, however, plays an important role in Calisthenics and is not just relegated to the back of the line. The majority of exercises described as calisthenic demand that the core be in place to keep the body's midline in place. If we exercise such as one that involves the front lever we will observe that while it's highly dependent on the strength of pulling your upper body part, but the core must keep the entire body straight , and also support all the leg weight. That means that a strong body that has been built by calisthenics is among the most robust you'll find.

As we have to build resistance in order to build strength, that means that we need to perform many of the more traditional core exercises to get rid of. However, this doesn't mean that the book doesn't include simple or less complex core exercises however, it does. it's not a reason to think that these alone aren't enough to rely upon to help build the level of strength that required to get to a higher standard.

The more advanced core workouts such as those you've never heard of previously, like the half lever are popular in gymnastics circles. They build such a strong core that once you've mastered them, they could make other core activities seem like child's play. There is no doubt that if you're able to master certain of the more difficult movements, you could fairly claim to possess one of the best cores.

THE SCAPULA

Forget large shoulders and wide backs, a person's ability of balancing and control their scapula is the primary source of strength in the upper body. The scapulas, also known as the shoulder blades, are the place where muscles and bones of the arms connect to the shoulder, and the scapula marks the place in which they join. In essence, the scapula capable of four actions that are protraction, fall, acceleration and retracting. When you slack your shoulders or turn your shoulders towards your ears, it is possible to elevate. Depression occurs when you make your shoulders drop to the bottom. Retraction happens when you pull your head back, and then expand your arms. when you round your back and shift your shoulder blades and spine away from each other, protraction occurs.

If the scapula could be made as strong as it is and you can build up the strength you gain within the body will be transmitted more efficiently. Of the many body parts that are that are involved in the movements of Calisthenics especially the more complex ones, it is the scapula that likely to be the most significant, but not well-known. The scapula contains the muscles of the rotator-cuff. which is described by Wikipedia as follows:

The muscles that make up the rotator-cuff are vital to shoulder movements as well as for maintaining the stabilization of shoulder joints. The muscles are derived from the scapula, and they connect to the back of the humerus creating a band around the shoulder joint. The humerus's head is held in the scapula's tiny and narrow glenoid fossa. The glenohumeral joints are similar to each other. described as a golfer's ball that is sitting on the golf tee.

The rotator-cuff muscles play multiple roles, including an abduction function, as well as internal and external rotation of the shoulder, while also stabilizing the glenohumeral joint and regulating the humeral head's translation. Infraspinatus and subscapularis are significant in abduction of the shoulder of the scapular plan producing forces up to three times more than that generated by the muscles of the supraspinatus. But, due to its time shoulder, it is the supraspinatus that tends to be better suited in the general abduction of shoulders. The anterior part of the supraspinatus tendon exposed to significant loads and strain, and performs its primary function.

If you're not a physiological athlete to the above, this description might appear to be a bit of rubbish, but the initial sentence is all we have to learn from it. The muscles of the rotator cuff are vital for shoulder movement and to ensure your shoulder's stability.

Your ability to perform the most challenging movements of Calisthenics depends on the capability of the rotator-cuff muscles in your body to stabilize your shoulder joint and allow the other muscles to perform the work. This includes pull-ups, frames and front levers, single-arm chin-ups and many more activities that require intense strength. In the section on mobility I will discuss a few exercises essential to improve shoulder health and should be performed by all regardless of your initial strength level.

STRETCH-ARM STRENGTH

Calisthenics, as well as a lot of gymnastics that extends puts a lot of emphasis on the phenomenon of straight-arm power. If you don't understand this term, you've likely seen it utilized. Gymnasts will use it on television to perform moves on still hoops like Iron Cross and Crucifix or when they demonstrate their skill using the planche.

Straight-arm strength is exactly as it sounds it is the force that an elbow that is locked was put into. This causes a lot of strain upon the arms and the connective tissues, such as the biceps and tendon of the biceps and also wrists and hands. Exercises like the planche that we'll discuss in depth later in the book, utilize straight-arm strength, which would be difficult , or even impossible to perform. This is the reason why the majority of gymnasts and coaches have large biceps however, they don't do the routine exercise that involves biceps curls. The stress on the muscle that is stretched causes it to be a significant increase strength and size as well as allowing for some of the most advanced exercises in calisthenics.

The great benefit of pulling straight with an arm that is straight can be that it creates the back robust. When the arms are straight, the back muscles will have to be working extremely hard to apply some force to the floor. This increases the strength in a manner that cannot be replicated in any other manner. This is the reason why gymnastics and calisthenics athletes have a strong back muscle. There are numerous exercises in this book that require straight-arm strength. Front lever, planche back lever, as well as the human flag are only a few of the movements that reveal this fascinating and unique element of Calisthenics.

TEACHING THE NERVOUS SYSTEM

A unique feature of Calisthenics is that the body's nervous system is being strengthened, and this can only be experienced performing intense exercises. While it isn't mentioned, it is more evident as the body being strained and stretched to the point that you feel like it's been working harder than the muscles you have.

This aspect of Calisthenics is best practiced in moves that require a lot of muscle groups at once or that require a lot of tension in the muscles to be maintained for long time. The most common causes of this are planche and the front and back levers as well as extremely complex movements such as the pull-up for one arm. It is likely that you are unable to keep doing these exercises over and over again because the body gets exhausted and fatigued after a short period of time. This is normal and only a sign that the exercise has done its job.

It is also seen in strength and conditioning, weightlifting and powerlifting. Imagine performing deadlifts of one rep maximum. A workout like this requires an enormous amount of energy generated that you can't keep doing it over and over and repeatedly. You might be able to do some reps, but your body will exhaust following that. This is the exact phenomenon that occurs during the high-level Calisthenics movements and is accomplished by using exercises using body weight.

Chapter 8: Benefits Of Calisthenics For A Quick Training

Calisthenics benefits of describing speed explained

It is a great way to get fit and running at the neck speed to win trophies and headlines. But, many athletes and runners who are quick to train believe that gym isn't required to increase speed. Some people believe that gymnastics training reduces your speed. This is not the reality. The following gymnastic advantages for speed training will be able to solve the issue nicely.

Offers a variety of workouts

One of the most beneficial aspects of training in gymnastics is that it allows for a variety of possibilities for your speed-training. By combining knee heights handles, crunches, handles and plates with a very short time between sets, it is assumed that your body will be as quick as is possible. Make sure you keep moving and experiment with various exercises to help get your body more fit.

Improves coordination

If you are discussing the benefits of gymnastics to speed training, it is important to not forget about coordination. The coordination of your body plays a major role in your speed and if your coordination is off, you won't be able to boost sales. Other runners can eventually smash you. However, if you are able to train in diverse gymnastics multiple times per week, you'll be more coordinated and , as a consequence you will speed up.

You get stronger

One of the biggest benefits of using gymnastics for speed training is that you're strengthening your body with every session. Of course, you have ensure that you're fueling up with nutritious food and drinks and you are getting enough rest. But when you practice gymnastics with braces and pushups, and every other exercise you typically do , it will make you more powerful and improves the strength of your body and speed.

You're probably convinced that you require calisthenics as part of your fitness program if you wish to increase your speed to the point that others, like Scouts, will observe. You do not want to rank as the slowest one on the field and you certainly don't want to finish second. You want to be the best which is why you practice every chance you get using all the techniques you've acquired to help you reach your goals of winning.

However, if you don't incorporate gymnastics to other equipment and equipment, you'll eventually hit your glass ceiling , and remain there. Instead, take advantage of the advantages of gymnastics in speed training and training , as the experts do. Calisthenics isn't "old class" or outdated, and it will definitely not hinder your progress. They will help you become more efficient, stronger, and more efficient than ever before. If you aren't convinced Try incorporating gymnastics into your routine , and you'll be sure to achieve all speed goals you set for yourself.

Calisthenic Training is the key to training success

There are many regimens, pills, and diets which can aid you in your fitness and health. Certain of them can help and motivate people, however some can trick you into quick-term results that don't result in the greatest fitness and health in the long-term.

Remember that when you are doing calisthenics, the most effective approach should include motivation, training regimen, and your diet.I will provide you with an overview of these three pillars to reaching your health and fitness targets in the long run.Let's begin by motivating yourself. When we are motivated, we are able to examine your beliefs as well as your mindset and the goals you have set for yourself. Naturally, goals are vital.

First, you must set goals to meet the desired goal. The benefits of exercise with weights are so evident that it is impossible to overlook the benefits, yet sometimes they happen. We put things off in our path. We allow other priorities take over our fitness and health. However, our fitness and health is a crucial aspect of our lives that can have positively impacted everyone else Aryans.

When you are setting objectives, you should consider the many important motives behind these goals. For instance, I want to lose 10 pounds, and I feel great about myself, or I walk 2 miles in order to keep up with my children and to be a great parent. Make your goals clear however, you must provide a solid reason to reach your targets. It is essential to keep the motivation to achieve them in your daily life.

You should also consider your mindset and your beliefs by motivating yourself.

Attitude is an important factor in what you're doing. If you don't have adequate access, you're probably not going to have the right actions. For instance, if you believe that you don't have the time to train in calisthenics then you're not right. Your attitude is wrong as well as your goals are muddled. Before you can ever change, you need to change your mindset.

If you aren't doing the right thing and don't achieve the desired results Take a look at the way you think. This is where you control your thoughts and not the reverse. You must take charge and your philosophies will help you in this.

The philosophy of the mind takes you to a higher level. You are able to choose your own philosophical beliefs and pick which beliefs you will accept. In my personal life, I hold an idea that training in calisthenics is an essential part of enjoyment and duty.

You must consider your beliefs, attitudes and objectives as you work towards your fitness and health goals.Another important aspect to consider is the importance of training. The most effective calisthenics workouts include three elements that include resistance training cardio weight training and the ability to stretch.

Calisthenic resistance training involves weight gain and is important for maintaining and increasing muscle tone and strength.Cardiovascular calisthenics exercises include fitness and weight gain and are great for burning body fat.Flexible training protects you from injury. It can help you maintain proper posture and move in every seam.

Nutrition is the third crucial factor. There's an abundance of information, and you aren't sure what you should accept. But, you don't wish to embark on diets, which are only a temporary solution. Learn about nutrition, and you will learn the best practices for healthy eating.

As I was beginning to build muscle I was thinking I should limit myself to push-ups, squirts and Squats for building muscle. Then I tried them. I became proficient at these exercises, and then I began to work out on the rig.

I have completed a variety of free-weight programs, and the majority of them were identical. I was in need of something fresh and more extensive.

It is vital to recognize the different kinds of body weight since every method can be utilized to serve a specific purpose. Simple physical exercises like pullups, pushups, and bodyweight squats could be utilized to build endurance and strength.

Training in calisthenics, however can be described as a cardio workout.

Since I am aging my cardio to an even pace that is why I often utilize body weight as well as other methods of training to supplement the need to exercise. However, aside from my dislike of the steady state of aerobic exercise also extremely important advantages of doing intense gymnastics to exercise:

One of the major advantages of Calisthenics is the improvement in endurance of the cardiorespiratory system that is the capacity of your body to absorb processes, release, and hold oxygen in order to produce the energy required to carry out an activity fully.

It is distinguished by a healthy and efficient lung and heart. Cardiorespiratory (cardio) endurance is more significant than the growth of muscles, but it is among the most under-appreciated elements of fitness.

If you're more able in your cardio, you will be able to effortlessly do more in a shorter time. This can improve your capacity to complete work, sports and other daily activities. By combining basic gymnastics and weight training, you will develop muscles as well as train your lung and heart.

This can help you do other physical exercises better. The majority of people are both tired and energized when they try to do simple tasks such as climbing stairs to lift boxes or trying to get the bus.

The activities are physically demanding and fitness tests. The gym is full of rats. get injured due to the fact that they are prone to fatigue. If your body is exhausted after a hard workout it's a sign of an insufficient healing.

Your muscles don't receive enough oxygen to allow for a complete recovery. Insomnia can cause poor posture and can lead to injuries that can be serious. In general, you'll be healthier if your lungs and heart become more healthy.

Through conditioning, you will effectively increase your capacity to live your life to the maximum. However there are many people who believe there's a particular "target the heart area" that can aid in burning fat and increase the endurance of your heart.

It is not true and this kind of zone doesn't exist. The athletes who have the greatest cardiovascular endurance - the balance of an active lung and heart condition and an athletic physique are those who do intensive exercises like sprinters.

In the end, it will take a while to last. Be aware that exercising for physical gymnastics is extremely intense and challenging. You must be constantly developing especially if you have spent much of your time after cardiovascular exercise that is published in a lot of magazines.

Calisthenics exercise example

Coach Lomax handles a vast range of gymnastics moves. Many of them you've seen or heard about, and some may have even performed previously. But a lot of them are brand new.

Here's a list of calisthenics that instructor Lomax will instruct you on:

Split jump

Jumping Jacks

Simulated skipping rope

Standing with a twist

Well, bend

windmill

High knees

Jogging in the street

marching

Calisthenics may appear easy to people who are not experts, but the secret is to practice them beforehand. Start by doing every exercise in a 60-second time frame, and after that, you can move onto the next move.This circuit workout is significantly more exciting and enjoyable than the traditional cardio exercise.

When you're proficient in these calisthenic basics Once you are comfortable, you can move on to moving to the Animal Calisthenics movement, which puts more emphasis on the lungs, the heart and muscles.

Six main reasons it is crucial to train for weights

Do you want a high-priced gym, and access to glittering machines, expensive equipment and magical powders to increase strength and health?

Training with weights is among the most flexible efficient, cost-effective, and economical methods of training available to professional athletes as well as non-professional fitness people.

Body weight exercises can be performed anywhere

There's no need to pay for a gym membership or costly equipment to take advantage of the physical fitness ... you've got everything you require right today.

Outside or inside ... There are numerous exercises for weight training can be done to increase your strength, fitness and endurance.

The Calisthenics program for body weight is the perfect way to begin.

If you're beginning an exercise program, resistance training is the ideal starting point to start.Gymnastics provides you for a physical base that allows you to efficiently and safely incorporate the most advanced exercises in your resistance.

Learn to manage your body weight prior to investigating other training methods.

Gymnastics with weights can be modified for every stage of fitness.There are a variety of ways of working out in a gym that utilizes the weight ... making it simpler or more challenging.

Thus, they're suitable for both experienced and novice fitness fans.

Bodyweight exercises that are based on naturally occurring body movement.Resistance training techniques usually are not able to directly improve movements that are commonly utilized in daily routine ... however, this isn't the case for bodyweight gymnastics.

The level of fitness is usually determined by your ability to control the movement in your own body ... rather than your capability to regulate the motion that an item.

Train in a way that you naturally move to experience more physical improvements that are in line with reality.

The use of body weight in gymnastics will increase strength and endurance, and strength

Based on the exercise used in the set-ups, reps and sets as well as the intensity ... You can gain strength, strength and endurance either individually or in combination.

The demands of sports and work are not always the same in one dimension ... instead, they are they are a mix of strength as well as endurance, strength, and endurance.

The gym is a fantastic opportunity to strengthen all three , and move smoothly from one strength to the next.

Training with body weights will increase strength and endurance to the heart in fat burning.When we are most likely to participate in a fitness program, we are looking to increase our strength and endurance of the cardiovascular system ... as well as burning off unwanted fat.

Gymnastics can perform each of these ... within the same session.

By adjusting the intensity of the intensity of your exercise, stress level and training intensity you can efficiently and effectively build strength, improve fitness and slimmer

Don't be deceived by the simple gymnastics that you can do with body weight ... they are one of the most effective methods to increase your strength and fitness.

It's not that it's difficult however, that does not mean that they're lightweight or useless ... Try one-arm push-ups or a one-arm pull-up on one leg if you're not convinced by me.

Weight training is the core of any fitness plan ... It's the perfect starting point and is a vital component of your fitness program as you progress to more exercises.

Chapter 9: Important Nutritional Principles

As with all exercise calisthenics should be coupled with a healthy and balanced diet to perform. Your body requires proper nutrition for proper functioning. Just being alive needs a certain amount of calories to provide energy to your brain, heart and the other organs that are vital to your health.

The amount of calories you require every day, even if do nothing but lie on your bed for the entire day is known as your Base Metabolic Rate, or BMR. There is a good chance you're BMR is the biggest portion of the calories you use up during the course of a single day. For some BMR is about 75% of calories burned in a single day.

The majority of BMR calculators use an equation that calculates both your weight and height. However, they're usually only estimations. Although your actual BMR is likely to lie in this spectrum, it's dependent on other variables like the temperature of your environment and genetics.

If you're working out to build musclemass, it's crucial to eat certain types of nutrients. This is due to the fact that, although the majority of our body cells are composed of the same substance that our muscles require quite much more of the same substances than other cells.

We'll go through nutrients fast. They are basically a source of nourishment that your body can't make by itself. Since we're not plants, which are able to create themselves food items, we have to eat to provide our body with these essential nutrients.

First, the nutrients that are
carbohydrates
. Carbs usually yield 4 calories per grams. Although carbs are often given negative reviews in fitness and diet programs, they are actually essential sources of energy within the body.

In fact, certain carbohydrates (called basic sugars) require minimal or no digestion, so they can be utilized by the body to generate energy. This is the reason you experience an energy boost after eating excessive sweets. There's simply too much energy available in your body and you get some sort of energy surge.

It is important to be mentioned that it's totally possible to follow the diet you want that is free of carbohydrates. The energy you require can come from other sources for instance, fats and proteins. While there are plenty of supporters of a carb-free diet however, it is important to do so cautiously. Since carbohydrates are the body's primary source in energy and energy expenditure, it could be risky to cut them out completely, particularly if you're working out for the first time.

Carb-free diets place your body into a state known as ketosis. This is a state in which your body, lacking energy-producing carbohydrates available to fuel itself, begins using fat reserves for energy. One of the results of this process is ketones. They are acidic and may be harmful to your body when they are at high levels.

If you want to completely avoid carbs the best option is to reduce the amount of carbohydrates you consume. It is also helpful to avoid the most basic carbs. Think of white bread, sugar white rice or anything that is processed in excess. These are foods that are regarded as having empty calories. They have calories, but they do not have much extra nutrition that comes from vitamins or minerals.

Instead, look for complex carbohydrates. They offer the added benefit of nutrition that isn't carbs, and are generally fuller as well. Complex carbohydrates are rich in fiber that your body is not able to process and thus is not utilized as calories however, it helps cleanse the digestive tract. However, they can also be digestible carbohydrates. Examples include whole wheat bread, rice that is not polished and roots crops like sweet potatoes.

The next type of nutrients are proteins

Similar to carbs, proteins provide around 4 calories per Gram. Proteins are comprised of building blocks known as amino acids.

They are crucial to living. They comprise 20 amino acid, of that are essential and can't be manufactured through the body.In particular proteins are essential in the creation as well as repair of tissue. If you recall the previous discussion, the process of muscle hypertrophy is basically the continual repair and development of muscle tissue. This is the reason why many diets for bodybuilding are rich in protein. Proteins are also what makes up your nails and hair.

High-protein foods are those that contain protein are fish, meat eggs, meat, milk, and milk-based products. There are numerous plant protein sources including beans (including soy) as well as nuts and grains.

Fats

There is another type of nutrients. Fats are a source of calories that range from 8-9 per grams. Although fat is often given the wrong treatment by people who are trying to lose weight, it's vital to consume small amounts. In the initial 20 minutes or so exercising, your body will use up your carbohydrate stores to generate energy. If you continue to work going, you'll be depleted of carbohydrate stores as your body begins to start processing fat available for metabolization. Fat can increase the absorption of fat-soluble Vitamins A D, E, and K.

There are a variety of kinds of fats that you can include that you can consume. Saturated fats can increase the level of low-density Lipoproteins (LDL). A high level of LDL are linked to an increased chances of suffering from cardiovascular problems like heart attack and stroke. Foods with high levels of LDL include meat fats butter, cheese, and milk products , as along with palm and coconut oils. One good guideline is the fact that saturated fats are typically solid at the temperature of room.

The other type of fat is the unsaturated type. This type of fat could actually aid in lowering your LDL levels and increase the levels of healthy cholesterol, HDL or high density lipoproteins. HDL which aid in removing LDL in your blood. This includes oils like olive oil, canola oil sunflower oil , and soy oil. Unsaturated fats are typically liquid at the temperature of room.

Vitamins

Another type of nutrient is those that is organic. There are 13 varieties of vitamins. They are necessary to normal body function and growth. Each vitamin performs a distinct role within the body. They are however divided in two categories: fat-soluble vitamins (ADEK) and the water-soluble vitamins.

Vitamins that are fat-soluble are more difficult to absorb since they require food fats (hence why it is not recommended to follow a strictly fat-free diet.) Vitamins that are water-soluble absorb better however they are more rapidly excreted via urine when the body isn't using them immediately.

Minerals

These are inorganic minerals that are required for the normal functioning of your body. Minerals essential to the body include potassium, calcium, iron and zinc.

They play a variety of roles within the body.

Finally,

water

is most likely the most crucial nutritional element. The majority the body constructed from water, and you are likely to be weak and weaker without it. It's even more crucial to drink plenty of water while exercising because you'll lose lots of water from sweat.

If you're exercising, you must to ensure that you are getting a balanced food balance. Diets high in protein are popular among those who are looking to build muscle. However, you must ensure that you're taking in enough other nutrients too.

If you are just beginning out it's not necessary to make major changes to your diet. It's important that you manage your portions and do not eat excessive amounts. It's tempting to eat lots particularly when you are exerting lots of energy during exercising. But, eating too much can make you exhausted in the short-term and will store excessive fat in the long run, and make all your hard work in vain.

You can have yourself evaluated by a nutritionist, if you enjoy. It can also be helpful to read labels on your food and compare them to your recommended daily allowance for each nutritional element.

In general, it is best to strive to eat in small portions of food, eating every 2 to 3 hours in order to maintain a healthy appetite. By limiting your food intake, it will lead you to eat more food when you sit down for a meal. Breakfast should be eaten no later than an hour after waking.

It is likely that your body has been for at least 8 hours without food. It is essential to replenish your body so that you can be energetic throughout the day. You should eat a snack about three to four hours after that, followed by lunch should be two to three hours later then another snack, and then, finally, dinner.

Avoid eating excessively processed foodsas they might be filled with empty calories or contain an high levels of fats that are unhealthy. Make sure you take enough water. Exercise can dehydrate you. Furthermore the muscle tissue is greater water content than fat tissues which means you'll require more to keep it in your body.

If you're not getting enough nutrients through your food, it might be worthwhile to consider taking supplements. Although you should be getting all the nutrients you need through the food you consume however, there are times when supplementation is required.

Remember that exercise and nutrition work in tandem. It's not practical and effective to focus on one without being attentive to the other. The best benefits if both complement one another.

Chapter 10: Top Tips Before Beginning

You may have been convinced to give calisthenics a go, but before you try anything else, bear on your toes that you must not attempt calisthenics with a weak heart. It is important to prepare your body and mind prior to doing all of the workouts you can find on the web. Be aware that calisthenics reduces the risk of sustaining an injury but if you decide to perform a rigorous callisthenic exercise with no prior experience and without the necessary endurance and strength of your body it is a matter of waiting for something to occur.

The most frequent error beginners make when they attempt to perform calisthenics is the exercises they perform aren't done correctly. There are numerous situations wherein people quit doing exercises or exercises after a couple of months due to failing to observe the effects of their efforts. It could be that the results required at the very least two more months to demonstrate the improvement which most people think, but this isn't the reality. The most important reason for their inability to perform is that they're performing the exercises incorrectly.

It is only a matter of time before you exhaust yourself doing 50 wrong pushups. Whatever number of sit-ups or pushups you complete, if are not doing it correctly, then you're just losing time and energy. It's better to complete only 5 push-ups performed correctly, than doing 20 improper ones. Make sure to control your muscular movements while doing these exercises. You will not create the muscles you desire if you're doing the wrong exercises.

Do a few basic calisthenic exercises at first. We'll discuss in a later chapter a series of easy exercises you can attempt for yourself. Try these easy exercises, and build up the sets gradually. Keep track of your improvements. If you believe that you've made progress, attempt to increase the intensity gradually. If you think that a specific part of your body requires more effort, you can include workouts in your routine to improve the strength of that particular area.

Keep in mind that the body you want is not going to be there the next day when you have began your workout. To achieve your goals, it might take time. Don't give up quickly if you don't observe your progress after a couple of days. Be patient and you will reap rewards. The celebrities you can see on the internet doing flawless calisthenics routines have years of experience to their credit.

If you're taking up calisthenics in order to shed weight, then it is important to incorporate diet into your diet and not only rely on exercises in callisthenics to shed the extra weight. Calisthenics is a way to build muscles and strength. It could be a great method of losing weight, doing it on its own won't be enough.

You should yourself discover the amazing benefits of calisthenics and how it can benefit your body and you. Keep yourself motivated by watching calisthenics videos and reading about related topics.

Chapter 11: The Press Ups and Dips

Dips and press ups are a great method to build strength in the upper and arm muscles as well as have the benefit of working the core, too.

Standard Press Up

For a normal press up, place yourself on the ground with arms stretched and shoulders wide apart. Your feet should be spaced shoulder-width apart, and you must maintain your balance using your feet. From here you can lower yourself to the floor using your elbows to bend. stopping when they reach an angle of 90 degrees. Return to the starting point for the final press-up. Your back should be straight throughout the workout.

Press Up Incline

You'll require an aerobics step or box to perform this workout. Start in the press-up position with your arms placed on the steps and feet planted on the floor. Lower yourself just as you would when you did press ups, but make sure that your back is straight. Return to your starting position for one repetition.

Decline Press Up.

The first step is to get the box or step aerobics. Make sure you are in the press-up position, with your legs resting on the box and your hands resting on the ground. Do a press-up at this point, making sure to keep your legs and back straight.

The Crossover Box is Pressing Up

You'll require an aerobics step or box to perform this workout. Set your left hand on the step, and the other on the ground . Then do a push-up in a way that ensures your chest is near to your step when you can. Once you are back to your starting point then switch your arms. Then "crossover" onto the opposite end of the blocks. You will then complete the same push up on the other side.

Diamond Press Up

For the Diamond Press Up, first begin by putting yourself into the Press-up position. Set your arms beneath your chest, your index fingers and thumbs overlapping to form the appearance of a diamond. Then, increase the width of your feet to assist with the balance. Lower yourself the same way as do a normal push up, but make sure at the bottom, your back is straight and your elbows point towards your feet.

Spider Press Up

Begin in the standard press-up position and complete the standard press up. While you lower your body to the ground, you can raise one knee and move it to the side until it touches your elbow. Reverse your body back to your beginning position and repeat the same exercise, changing legs for the next repetition.

Staggered Press Ups

Beginning in the normal pressing up posture, shift one hand slightly ahead of the other hand and do a press up. Once you've completed the set then switch arms and then repeat.

Bench Dip

To do the bench dip, you must first take a seat on a bench, or chair. After that, by supporting your weight using your hands, push yourself forward until you're not on the chair anymore. Then, lower yourself until the elbows form a an angle of 90 degrees. Then, raise your body back to finish the set.

The Bench is elevated. Dips

You'll need two chairs or benches for this workout. For the first time, begin by getting in the position of a bench dip and then place your feet on the opposite bench or chair, so that your legs are raised. You can dip like you normally and ensure that you are able to keep the legs in a straight position.

Chest Dips

You'll need parallel pars to complete this exercise however, two chairs may be used. Start with the bars in place and then stepping off of the floor by either jumping or bent your knees. By securing yourself with only your arms and drop yourself down until the elbows are at an angle of 90 degrees towards the ground. Then slowly raise yourself up making sure to keep your knees straight while you go. Lean slightly forward during this exercise to maintain your equilibrium.

One Arm Bench Dip

Starting in your dip, extend your right arm as well as your left leg to be level with the floor. Lower yourself, maintaining your leg and arm straight. Re-lift yourself change body positions and repeat the exercise until you have completed one rep.

Incline Dip

You will require two bars or chairs for this workout. Begin by putting your weight on your arms, then bringing your knees up to the chest. Make sure your legs are in line with the ground. Begin to lower yourself till your elbows are 90 degrees while leaning forward in order to maintain equilibrium.

Chapter 12: Following up with A Healthy Lifestyle And Diet

You've completed your entire routine of Calisthenics and cannot wait for the next one. The next day, and you feel the muscles in your legs and arms are aching. What can you do?

The importance of a proper pace and Rest

Many beginners jump into exercise with the belief that the more quickly they go through the exercises, the more quickly they'll achieve their desired fitness level. While there's no harm in wanting to get results, it is important to remember that your body requires to be monitored and rested in a manner that is appropriate.

If you are achy and exhausted after just a few hours working on your body's fitness, you may want to rest for a while. It is possible to continue your routine with stretching and warm-up exercises, or even reducing the amount of sets to 5 percent. In this means that your body is gradually exposed to the work you'd like it to perform.

Be patient with yourself and concentrate on completing the proper form for every exercise done correctly. It is important to focus on quality positions, not just the amount of sets and repetitions you can do within a single day. If you are attentive to the body's needs and giving yourself the relaxation time, you'll be more prepared to tackle every Calisthenics workout routine.

The right fuel is available

Human body can be an incredible machine. But, like trains or cars it requires the right type of fuel to function properly. It is impossible to finish an Calisthenics exercise and expect to reap all the benefits when you don't provide your body nutritious diet.

If you're unable to lift yourself up when doing push-ups or chin-ups it is possible to reduce your intake of foods high in carbs and sugars. Concentrate on getting fiber from fruits and vegetables as well as protein from meats and fish. Remove any sweets from your diet and you'll soon be capable of lifting and pushing your body effortlessly.

There are many diets recommended by nutritionists and fitness experts. In the days off it is possible to go to the library or a bookstore and pick up a couple of books to learn more about the ideal diet for you.

Get rid of the bad habits

Another crucial step to follow up on your exercise routine is to eliminate all your negative routines. It will require time and effort, however, if you begin to eliminate one habit that is harmful this morning, you'll be able to guarantee that the other ones will be removed in the coming time. Eliminate smoking and drinking too much. They'll do nothing to assist you in getting the Greek god-like body that you've always wanted.

Ready for the Challenge

Once you've completed the fundamental Calisthenics exercises You will surely be looking to improve their level of difficulty. Here are some suggestions on how to boost the Calisthenics workout routine.

1. Elevated Push-ups

It is done using your feet placed on a more elevated surfaceand then executing the push-up technique starting there.

2. Sustained Chin-ups

When you have reached the top of the bar, it is possible to stay in the position for five more seconds before dropping your body. It is possible to increase the time you take and the amount of repetitions you need to perform, to adapt the intensity of the exercise to the body's demands.

3. Leg Raises

This workout is difficult, and requires professional supervision. Instead of lifting your chin toward the bar it is expected to raise your legs and curl them towards your body. Then let your feet touch the bar.

4. V Sit-Ups

It is done by lying on a smooth surface and then moving your upper body towards your knees while lifting both legs up to the extended posture. Your body must resemble an V-shaped letter.

Chapter 13: The Key Training Principles to Ensure the best results

One of the key principles that is essential to any training program is "Progressive Overload.". This is simply the process of getting more and more difficult as time passes. This is the most important principle of training that has to be implemented to meet your objectives.

As you gradually increase the demands on the musculoskeletal system you're overloading and forcing your body to adjust. Due to the constant overload, you will increase your strength, build muscle mass and boost your endurance.

If you've been training in the gym for many decades and years, but have seen no progress then you're not applying the correct amount of overload.

If the demands you place on your muscles decrease with the course of time i.e. you cease working out or your exercise becomes more easy the muscles will atrophy (become shrinking) and you'll decrease your strength. This is referred to as reversibility.

How do you implement progressive overload?

The most popular method we'll encounter at gyms involves lifting more and heavier weights as time passes. But, if we're exercising without weights, it is necessary to apply progressive overload using various techniques.

There are a variety of methods for advancement, far beyond the boundaries of this guide. We'll be focusing on a handful of basic ones that will be most beneficial to you during your calisthenics training journey.

Example

If you do 10 push-ups during your exercise routine, you'll increase your strength while your muscles develop due to this. After a few weeks, performing 10 push-ups becomes simple since your body has adapted to the load. If you continue to do 10 push-ups per workout, you won't notice any additional results since your body doesn't have any reason to change -

it will handle the load with the way it is. Instead, you should apply the progressive overload repeatedly and repeatedly to get more outcomes.

To build more strength, endurance or muscle To increase your endurance, strength or muscle using one of the following techniques.

1. Progression 2: Increase Strength By Changing the Exercise

Through weight training it is simple to add weight to the bar. Through bodyweight training it is necessary to increase the resistance in by another method. It is important to gradually progress towards harder and more difficult exercises.

For instance for example, in the push-up series, you'll gradually progress to do wall push ups to one-arm push-ups. Squatting exercises begin by doing basic half squats up to pistol squats. These exercises require greater strength than the earlier exercises.

The best exercise progressions will be outlined on the progression charts in the next chapter.

Progression 2: Resets Increased

Another way to increase your increase your workload is simply to perform more repetitions. If you can perform five push-ups, you can increase the number to 6 7 8, 9, and 10. You can progress to 20 or fifty or 100 reps depending on the goals you have set.

To maximize your strength gains, it is recommended to do three sets that are 3-8 repetitions, with 90 to 180 seconds of rest between sets. When you are able to complete three sets of eight reps in an exercise, then you can move to a more challenging exercise.

To maximize muscle growth, you should aim for five sets of six to 12 reps , with 60-120 seconds of rest between sets. Once you reach the upper portion of this range, you need to move to a harder exercise.

For maximum endurance gains, it is recommended to do 5- 10 sets that consist of more than 12 reps , with the rest period of 0-60 seconds between sets.

It's important to keep in mind that these ranges are only rough guidelines. It is possible to gain muscles mass in the 3-8 rep range but it's not as effective as 6-12 reps.

If you are looking to increase your strength and endurance, muscle mass, and strength I suggest working on the strength range to start with for at the least 8 weeks before shifting to the muscles mass range for 8 weeks and finally the endurance range for eight weeks.

The Progression 3 is to Increase the Volume

The third way of progressing is to increase volume. Volume is defined as the set multiplied by reps, then multiplied by resistance. It is possible to do more sets of the exercise, or add additional exercises that target the same muscles groups to increase the volume.

For instance, you could go from three set of 10 repetitions push-ups to five sets of 10 push-ups.

You can add three set of dips for body weight to boost the quantity.

4. Progression: Increase the frequency of training

The fourth way to increase overload is increasing the training frequency. For example, instead doing a muscle workout every week, you can do it twice or three times each week.

This technique is very effective when you have a particular desired strength goal or weaknesses.

Many newbies make the error of training too frequently because they believe that training more will result in more outcomes. This is not the case.

In reality, there's an "sweet place" in training.

The body may become weaker temporarily after a hard training session. It is important to allow for enough recuperation before you can train again. This allows you to get stronger and move toward your fitness and health objectives, which we'll discuss in the following article.

It's just the same as not exercising enough. For this calisthenics training program we will be using three times a week as a good starting point. Actually, you could attain a very high level with this training frequency.

Long-term consistency is more important than short-term intensity.

Progression 5: Reduce Rest Intervals

The fifth way to achieve gradual overloading is to decrease the amount of work between sets. This means you're doing exactly the same work but in shorter amounts of time. You can go from a rest period of 120 seconds from 90 seconds to 60 seconds and then 30 seconds.

Chapter 14: The Components In An Exercise Program

Six components are included in the workout routine. Although each one of them may be described with a different title, the components are identical.

These are the components:

1)Warm up

2)Stretching

3)Cardio training

4)Muscular training

5)Cool down

6)Stretching

It is essential to recognize that every step needs to be done. There are many people who don't perform each of these steps regardless of the reason, and by doing this, they significantly increase the risk of injuries. A lot of people don't stretch , or they do it just for a short time, which causes them to be forced to stop exercising.

1)Warm up

Your warm-up should be a slow, rhythmic aerobic exercise that involves all major muscle groups like your legs. The warm-up is a way to prepare for your body for greater intensity exercise. The lower intensity warm-up is recommended to last at minimum five minutes. It should be completed before doing any other exercise.

2)Stretching

The type of stretching described here is extremely low-intensity and is designed to stretch specific muscles. Each stretch posture is recommended to be performed for between 20 and 30 seconds, and you should stretch your muscles daily.

3)Cardio training

The aim of cardio-training is to perform a variety of aerobic exercise, such as walking, jogging, climbing stairs, etc. and at 80percent of your maximum heart rate.

You can determine your rate of heart by measuring your heart rate, then subtracting away your age. So if your heat rate of 210 degrees and you're 30 years old, 180 x 210 = 30. To reach the 80% rate of your heart will need to be the 154th percentile. The cardio training process also involves burning calories from 65percent from your rate upwards so when your heart rate hits at 127, you're starting to burn fat.

Training in cardio should be performed three times a week for around 30 minutes per session. Consider the chores you perform in your home every day since they will be easily incorporated in this framework, meaning there could not be a need to perform anything else as a separate task.

4)Muscle training

Training for muscle can be completed by using weight machines or not and, if the exercise requires free weights, they can be items found around your house. Training for muscles should be done at a minimum of 20 minutes, two - three times per week.

5)Cool down

The cooling down is crucial and is a low-intensity aerobic exercises that aid your body in returning to its pre-exercise condition. The cool-down should be performed in conjunction with your workout routine and take no less than 3 minutes.

6)Stretching

The last set of stretches is to simply stretch muscles to prevent becoming stiff and painful. If you are doing any kind of training with bodyweights, the focus is on the quality of your workout, not the quantity.

Growing too large

Many who start exercising think that their muscles will become too large for the goals they're trying to accomplish However, this is extremely unlikely since it takes time and dedication to get muscle mass that looks like bodybuilders. To appear this way , you'll have to exercise six days per week for a minimum of four hours every day. You must be working hard to strengthen your muscles.

Chapter 15: What Are The Advantages Of Calisthenics

You can be sure there are a lot of benefits that come with this particular type of exercise which is why it's recommended to consider these to prove that this kind of exercise is one you ought to consider doing. As you can see, calisthenics will benefit both your body and you in a variety of ways.

You do not require any equipment.

This is the most significant benefit from this kind of exercise is that it is not necessary to purchase the latest equipment to increase your strength and to work on those muscles. All you need is you and a program of exercise that we will go over in the future and you're good to go.

We should also be aware that you may be interested in investing in a pull-up bar that is placed through your doorway, as it allows you to perform one of the most essential exercises.

It increases your heart rate.

Like any other exercise one of the most important factors you must strive to accomplish is to increase your heart rate , and calisthenics is a great way to do this. But in the same way, it isn't able to raise it in the same way as other cardiovascular exercises however it is enough to have an impact. If you break into a little of a sweat and you feel slightly exhausted that you're doing the right thing with your workout routine, and you should try to do this throughout the day.

You become more flexible.

Because of the manner the various exercises that make up calisthenics stretch your abilities to the limit This means that you will become much more flexible. Naturally, due to the manner in how strength can be developed through various exercises, this means you get stronger , but your flexibility is not diminished.

There's another benefit to this. The more strong you get as you grow, the more flexible become. This leads to being able to perform more exercises for longer periods of time and also your flexibility being enhanced. So, you join this intriguing circle that allows you to gain from your workout in many ways.

It helps you lose Weight.

Calisthentics is also proven to assist people in losing weight, and the method by how it does this is fairly simple. Because it raises the heartbeat, it means that it boosts the rate of metabolism. Since you're burning energy the body will be looking to burn fat to replenish the depleted reserves. As consequently, you'll shed weight.

There's a second benefit to getting your metabolism up through exercise and that is that it means that your body will to burn more calories, even while resting. That is, it prevents you from putting on weight if you are mindful of what you eat , of course.

It's easier on your Joints.

Calisthenics is proven to be gentler on joints when compared with other types of exercise. There's just not the similar amount of stress and strain placed on your joints, specifically when compared to weightlifting, which means there is less chance to suffer injuries. Keep in mind that you are doing what was handed to you naturally, which means your body will recognize that it is stressed but you will not be pushing it to the limit at any time.

It certainly builds strength.

When you lift the weight of your body and lifting your own body weight, you'll be building strength. But the most important thing is that you're actually strengthening your body in a natural manner and, of course the body isn't likely to experience any more stress or strain that it was built to do. Also, it is completely safe to build up strength.

It is also important to note that apart from strength, it will boost your endurance levels, which can lead to being in the same circle described in the article about your flexibility.

It allows you to work on Your Balance.

Because of how the exercises are conducted and the method by which the exercises are designed It is likely that you'll get an evenly-paced workout that works with different muscles over the duration of an exercise set. By focusing on the various muscles in a balanced manner, it will result in their strength developing in a consistent manner and will benefit your physiology when compared to other forms of exercise.

It improves coordination.

In order to reap the benefits from all the exercises, it's necessary for that you are able to execute various functions and move in a coordinated manner. You can improve your capacity to perform your movements in a particular manner, and without the capability to do this, it is impossible for you to successfully complete an array of excrcises. A lack of coordination could result in an increase in the chance of injury.

It can be done anywhere and at any time.

This could be the most significant benefit of calisthenics because it can be performed anywhere and it is not dependent on what you're doing at the moment. This is due to its non dependence on equipment since it's entirely about yourself and the way you move. It basically means that when you learn calisthenics, there is no excuse anymore for you to not working out to get stronger and fitter each day.

Chapter 16: The importance of Calisthenics for a simple training

Calisthenics: explaining the importance of speed

Calisthenics is great to shape your neck and provides the speed needed to win the trophies and caps. But some speedy athletes and runners think that gymnastics do not have to be speeded up. For some, when a baby grows, it will grow. This could not be further than the reality. The following gymnastics benefits of speed training will help solve this issue.

There are some changes to your education.

One of the most beneficial aspects of training in gymnastics is the fact that you will experience many different options for your routine. If knee heights and gloves, crumbs and plates are combined with no rest between seats, think that your body will be as quick as it can be. Be sure to keep working hard and do various exercises to make your body in shape.

You'll be able to better coordinate your activities.

When discussing the advantages of gymnastics that are fast-paced and you don't want to lose focus on coordination. The coordination of your body plays a major role in the speed at which you're and if your coordination isn't fluid, you won't be able to increase sales. Other runners may eventually turn your off. If you practice various gymnastics at least once each week, you'll perform better in coordination and as a consequence you will speed up.

You'll be extremely strong.

One of the obvious advantages of speed training is the strength you gain every time you do an exercise. Make sure that you have sufficient energy for healthy drinks and food, and get ample rest, but if perform bra and villi gymnastics, as well as all the other exercises you normally do during training, you will get stronger and improve your power and speed.

I'm sure you'll agree that you should incorporate calisthenics into your program of training to establish the speed that can be seen by others, which includes Scouts. You do not want being the slowest one working in your field and you certainly don't like to rank second. You're determined to be successful therefore you'll be prepared every time you have the chance using all the techniques you've learned to reach the goals you've achieved.

If you don't include aerobics into the other equipment, you'll reach an unattainable ceiling and stay there. Instead, you should shift your focus towards positive aspects of life, like training and building muscle.

Calisthenics isn't "old old school" or outdated , and won't hinder your progress. They actually make you more efficient, stable, and faster than you have ever been. If you don't believe you can benefit from aerobics, consider incorporating it in your routine and feel certain that you can meet every speed goal you set for yourself.

Calisthenic Training: The Role In Successful Training

There are many supplements, exercises and diets that can help you improve your fitness and health. Some are helpful and motivate people, while some will trick you into believing that they can provide immediate results that will not result in better health and wellbeing over time.

Be aware that when it comes to gymnastics an effective approach must include exercise, motivation and a healthy diet. I'll give you the three essential elements for achieving your long-term wellness and health goals. Let's begin by motivating yourself. If you are motivated you are able to look at your approach, your philosophy and goals. Goals are of course essential.

First, you must set the goal of achieving this. The advantages of weight training calisthenics are so obvious, it's hard to overlook the benefits, but it isn't always easy to remember.

We put things off the road. We let other benefits enhance our health and fitness. But our health and abilities are an integral part of our lives and can have a positive effect on the rest of Aryans.

When you set goals, focus on several reasons that you achieve the goals. For instance, I shed 10 pounds, and I feel great about my body, or I run 2 miles to continue to be with my kids and be a good mother. Make your goals clear however, you must offer a strong reason to reach the targets. It is essential to keep the highest level of motivation throughout your day.

It's helpful to look at your philosophy and attitude with a sense of motivation.

Attitude is the genesis of your actions. If you're not using the correct attitude then you're not taking the right actions. For example, if think that you don't have enough time to train for calisthenics you're wrong. It's not the right approach which means your priority is muddled. Before you decide to make a change, you need to change your perspective.

When you're doing things wrong, and you're not receiving the results you want take a look at how you're thinking. You have control of your thoughts rather than the opposite. You must take charge and your mindset can help you do this.

Philosophies go beyond the surface. You have the option of choosing your choice of philosophy and then decide on the beliefs you believe in. In my personal life, I hold an idea that gym training is crucial for both task as well as joy.You should consider your attitude, philosophy and goals in achieving your fitness and health objectives. Another important factor is to train. The most effective gymnastics exercises comprise three components such as cardiovascular training for strength and flexibility.

Resistance training for Calisthenics is all focused on gaining weight and is vital for maintaining and enhancing the strength and tone of muscles. Cardiovascular gymnastics is a form of fitness that can lead to weight loss and are excellent to lose fat in the body. The flexibility of your training can help protect you from injuries. It helps maintain your proper posture and move across all layers.

Nutrition is the third crucial aspect. There's an abundance of information, and you aren't sure which supplements to use. You do not wish to stick to a diet, which is only a quick fix. Learn about food, and you will learn the best practices for healthy eating.

When I first started to train to increase my weight, I was thinking I'd have to perform push-ups and splashes, and squats to build building muscle. So, that's what I did I did very well with these exercises, then I made the team.I tried a variety of free weight loss programs, but the majority of them were identical. I wanted something different and more thorough.

It is essential to differentiate between different types of bodyweight as any type of method can be utilized for a specific goal. Simple physical exercises like stretching, push-ups and bodyweight squats are utilized to build the strength as well as general health.

Training in California is, in contrast is not just an aerobic workout.As I age with my heart, I will continue to employ bodyweight as well as other methods of training to satisfy the requirement for a cardiovascular diet. Apart from the issue with cardio while in a stable location, there are also positive aspects to the intense workout of gymnastics as a type of cardio.

One of Calisthenics greatest benefits is its improvement in endurance in the cardiovascular system, which is your body's capability to process, capture release and store oxygen in order to carry the required energy to complete a task ultimately.It is distinguished by a well-functioning and healthy lung and heart.

The cardiovascular (cardio) endurance likely more crucial than losing fat or muscle growth, however it's among the most overlooked aspects of fitness.

If you are able to resist more in your cardio, you will be able to easily train for more frequently. This can improve your ability to perform sports, work and everyday life. If you mix the basics of gymnastics with weight-training it will help you build your muscles as well as train your lungs and heart.

This can help you do other activities that require physical effort better. Many people get overwhelmed and exhausted when they tackle simple tasks like collecting boxes on the steps or trying to get on the bus.These tasks require physical fitness and testing for fitness. A lot of rats at the gym get injured due to the fact that they get tired quickly. When your body gets tired after a long day of exercise it's a sign of a slow healing.

Your muscles aren't getting the proper amount of oxygen to fully recover. The result is a bad shape which then results in personal injuries. In general, you'll be more healthy in the event that your lungs and your heart are healthy.

By focusing on conditioning, you'll be able to dramatically improve your capacity to live until the very end. However there are many people who believe there's a particular "target heart region" that can help you reduce fat and increase the endurance of your heart.

This is not the case and there isn't any such zone. The athletes with the highest cardiac endurance - that is, a balance between the health of your lung and heart function as well as physical fitness that is functional are those who perform intense exercise, like sprinters.

In essence, it will be a matter of time. But, keep in mind that the physical training for gymnastics is extremely intense and demanding. It is essential to continue learning particularly if you have were primarily in cardio classes, and are featured in a lot of magazines.

A good illustration of California practice

The Lomax trainer handles a wide variety of gymnastics movements. You've heard of some and may have seen them in the past. However, a lot of you are turning green.

Here's a list of chestnut exercises you can do. Coach Lomax will teach you:

* Division jump
* Cranes that jump
* Simulation skipping rope
* Stable rotation
* Loop and reach

* windmill
* Knee-high
* Running on site
* marching

The Calisthenic exercises may appear easy to people who are not experts, but they must to be planned ahead. Start by taking 60 seconds to complete each exercise before you go to the next stage. The circular workout can be more enjoyable and thrilling than a typical kind of cardiovascular workout.If you're comfortable in these calisthenics basics You can begin with this Animal Calisthenics movement, emphasizing the heart, lungs and muscles.

A COMPLETE WORKOUT PROGRAM FOR BEGINNERS and advanced professional with A PROCESS AND TIPS FOR YOUR training

There isn't a universal fitness program for newbies because everybody is different. But, there are some guidelines to keep in mind while exercising to adapt quickly. If you decide to begin your fitness journey this will be beneficial to you. It's the right time to start fitness and it's never too late to get started. It's important to follow the first steps in starting with a fitness routine. Let's look at these steps.

Step 1: Speak to your doctor.

This is vital since when you sit down for a long time, you aren't likely to engage in activities that could harm your. Before starting, ensure that you are in good physical shape to determine if exercise that is strenuous is an inconvenient.

Step 2: Begin with a slow pace.

Health is the main motive to engage in an exercise routine. If you are sitting for a long period of time and do not work out for two hours that first day. You'll be embarrassed and might even harm yourself, therefore you shouldn't take a break for a few minutes which is why you stop. So, any fitness program for newbies should be simple.

But don't roll. As you advance your body's body will adjust quickly and you can alter your pace.

Step 3. Include the appropriate items in your fitness program for people who are just beginning.

If you are just beginning the process, you might want to start with just one tour. A minimum of five to 10 minutes in the beginning of your day is an ideal way to start.

While you move through your program of training, include stretching exercises, strength warm-up, warm-up and cool down so that you don't get injured. It's not a risk. Start by setting simple objectives, like taking 10 minutes a day to run. From there, you can increase your efforts. The goal is to complete at minimum 20 minutes of physical activity every day, but ideally one hour.

4. Always be sweaty

Be careful not to get too active when exercising. Your aim should be to run each day for between 20 and 30 minutes. It is also important to speak to others in the course of your activities however, not in a quiet manner. Also you should take some breath while exercising.

Step 5: Turn off the device.

As your body becomes accustomed to specific types of exercise the body becomes more efficient and efficient, meaning that should you continue to do the same training method your intensity will diminish.

Thus, when you do your workouts every day, switch your strength and cardiovascular exercises. For instance, on the next day, you might opt to exercise for cardiovascular as well as a four-strength bicycle. The following day, it could be a good time to take a break from cardiovascular workouts and do you can do a push-up to strengthen your muscles. Remember to keep your intensity up regardless of what you do.

6 Step: Eat healthy Drink plenty of water and rest.

There is no exercise program that will make you be more attractive and healthier, if you're not performing it correctly and drinking enough water and getting enough rest. A majority of people need more than 8 hours of rest each day.

Your diet should consist of high in protein lean as well as complex carbohydrates, vegetables, fruits and healthy fats that are saturated. This means the elimination of refined carbohydrates, unhealthy food items such as sugar, and so on.

If you have been training for less than a year , and are looking to build muscle you could be considered an beginner. One of the most difficult things for newbies to build and build a body is to make sure that the program you are using for muscle building is well-designed. So, examine the initial bodybuilding program follow it and you'll soon be on path in building your physique and progressing towards more challenging applications.

The best thing about beginning the process of building muscle is that you'll probably get the most effective and speediest results within the first six or 12 months (if you follow the correct plan). This is a great moment, and you'll notice a shift within your body and your self. Follow the guidelines below, and give yourself three months, and you'll see huge gains. The only problem is that there's no alcohol. It's going to be hard to master, but if you're determined to be a hard worker it will pay off.

MUSCLE ROUTINE for Beginners

Beginners is able to follow a workout routine to achieve a perfect body shape, but not necessarily grow the size and muscle mass. The exercise for every muscle group will ensure that all muscles get familiar with the exercise that builds muscles. Before starting the workout, one should ensure that it is properly warmed up across the entire body. The warming session lasts about. 15-20 minutes. Some examples of these are walking, running, or running. These activities stimulate the muscles and help them prepare for exercise.

Training for the triceps

Double triceps dips

* The two rods are fixed against the other using the palms. The body is held in place by gluing it to the rail.

* Slowly bend and slightly bend to help support your back. It is recommended to

remain standing in the same position some time.

Repeat the process.

Work the triceps

* Position yourself in front of the pulley , and join the rod.

Attach the clamp to the weighed and keep the bar in place from above using both hands

• Slide the tray downwards and slowly lift it up

Extend the Barbel landscape

* One is located on a bench in the back

* The barbell is kept in hand, with hands raised.

Bend your elbows slowly to observe the bow movement and then hold the barbell an inch higher than your forehead.

• Return back to your previous position.

Training for biceps

Bicep curls

* Stand up

* Place the barbell weights in the appropriate place,

* Put the barbell on your shoulders, then slowly lower it.

Bicep curls that are sloping

• Sit down on the bench

Make sure you hold dumbbells in each hand.

* Lift one dumbbell to the level of your shoulders.

* Delay

* Repeat the process for the opposite side.

Barbells for concentration curls

This is among the most well-known and useful exercises using dumbbells for both genders.

• Sit upright on a couch or chair with your legs separated and an arm on the right part of the right.

Make a slight bend so that the elbow of your right fits comfortably within your right leg.

Use your left forearm to sit on the right side of your thigh

* Place the bar in your right hand , so that it is pointed towards you.

Put your right hand over your knee to keep your balance throughout the exercise.

The biceps workout begins with a gradual turning of the left forearm towards the shoulders. Concentric curls require that you focus on the biceps muscles, and make sure that your arm muscles are engaged.

The most effective exercise for shoulder muscles. Large shoulders can create an illusionary body. Everybody who is a strong-arm bodybuilder always gets extremely high marks in symmetry round. Also, you appear more powerful than you. This book I'm trying to present the best exercises for your shoulder muscles.

Front Layers

Barbell presses are an excellent method to build the first muscle of your deltoid. You can perform them at the blacksmith or on grass. By standing on the side of the sofa, raises the upper and middle back. Since these areas must be able to support shoulders and the upper body while working. Barbell pressures that maintain tension in the muscle of the deltoid.

This workout targets the deltoid muscles. The most effective way to perform this is to move the sides of the barbells. You can grasp something in one hand, and then lift the barb with the other until it's in line with the floor. Tilting eases pressure in your neck, and decreases and keeps pressure in the region where you're trying to focus. You can also utilize side branches using dumbbells. If you decide to add weight, your shoulder should be a little less from the ground to ensure that tension is maintained throughout the body throughout the entire time and to ensure that you don't fall during the exercise.

Chapter 17: Calisthenics Equipment For Home Use

We have discussed our belief that calisthenics is a sport that does require no equipment, and we stand by our assertion. Yet, in spite of the large range of possible exercises there are a few which can be benefited by using a budget equipment for calisthenics.
Pull-Up Bar

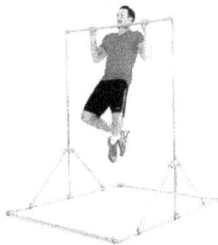

If you are using equipment for calisthenics The pull-up bar is the obvious option. You can find it in our calisthenics basics section, the push-ups are usually considered to be one of the fundamental exercises. Many consider them an entry point to fitness workouts worth doing!

You can either buy a pull-up bar to use at the home, use it at the gym, or go to the local park and utilize the goal posts, you should consider the pull-ups your first choice.

Ab Wheel

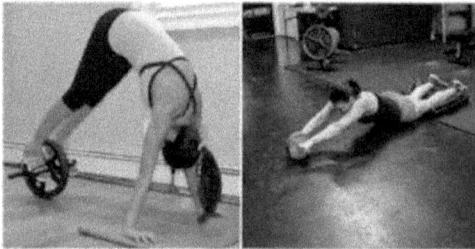

Although calisthenics is an all-encompassing exercise, there's no harm in focusing on the fundamentals of of your calisthenics exercises, especially when you consider the role it plays in helping the rest of your body.

Ab wheel exercises are the ideal method to achieve this. It targets not only the majority of abdominal muscles with a few sets, it also helps strengthen the shoulders, arms and chest as well as lower back as well.

It is possible to purchase one online for only $8, which isn't too bad given the amount of usage you'll get from it.

Skipping Rope

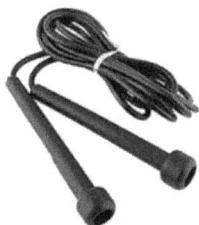

A skipping rope being part of your equipment for calisthenics might seem odd however, trust us.

The most important thing to know about calisthenics for beginners is that it's vital to have a solid warm-up. Without a proper warm-up it is not just your performance be affected and your safety be compromised too.

What better way to begin warming up than by using a skipping rope? It's a lot less expensive than a treadmill, and adds to an exciting and thrilling cardiovascular workout. Absolutely, nobody has time to complain about the opportunity to shed extra pounds ...

The skipping rope an cheap equipment that can offer you a challenge as you warm up. Take advantage of it as a chance to work hard.

Resistance Bands

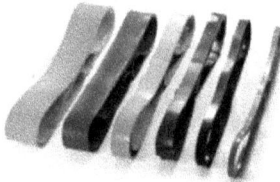

6 Levels

We are unable to imagine any more versatile piece of equipment for calisthenics. You can utilize virtually resistance bands to assist or test you with any beginner's calisthenics workouts!

For instance, if you're struggling doing push-ups, connect one of them to the bar and then hold the other end between your legs to enhance your posture.

In addition, if you were performing triceps dips then you can put an elastic band around your shoulders to add weight to your workout.

Resistance bands are on the lower portion on the exercise equipment range and can help improve your flexibility and shape.

Gymnastic Rings

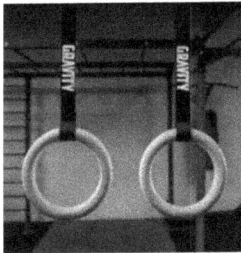

They're extremely difficult to use and should not be attempted by those who are new to calisthenics. But, everyone is unique and may be able to benefit by adding them to their calisthenics equipment list at the beginning of their training.

Rings for gymnastics are a challenge and I'm not trying to hide the fact. If you utilize rings for push-ups or for other exercises your muscles will find the workout to be more difficult than the typical bar pull-up.

This is due to the fact that the rings move in different directions and their stabilizers require to be used twice in order to help balance your body.

The benefit is that, with a lot of practice, you will be able to improve the balance and strength you have before and also prepare yourself for the most challenging exercises of calisthenics.

Parallette

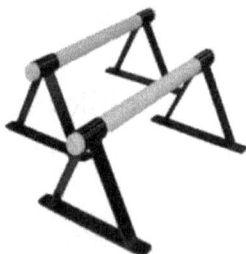

Have you ever wanted to create your perfect handstand? With Parallette it's far simpler than you think due to the fact that they take lots of stress from your wrists.

There are two kinds of parallels. The bigger ones are designed for exercises like tricepsand biceps, while smaller ones are used to be used for handstands and pushups.

The smaller ones function similarly as those resistance bands. They are able for hand support, or for more challenging hand push-ups through introducing an expanded range of movement.

These are great ideas for anyone looking to practice these exercises in the at-home comforts of their home.

Power Tower

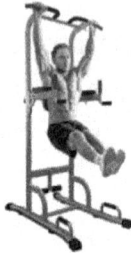

While it's costly in comparison to other equipment for calisthenics however, the potential for it to change your fitness and performance is not unattainable.

What is this mysterious power tower?

It is the equipment that is used to perform the chin-ups, push-ups and sit-ups and triceps dips as well as knee raises and many more. It is the most effective equipment for calisthenics beginner athletes, specifically because of its emphasis on the use of the body's weight during exercises.

Chapter 18: Advanced Calisthenics

The process of progressing is vital to increase the strength, endurance and power as well as mass. It's the most strenuous exercises that aid in building a stronger and ripped body. When you begin to notice an exercise that is easier for beginners than before, it's time to advance into the next step. Here are some difficult calisthenics workouts that you can incorporate into your routine to raise your challenge degree.

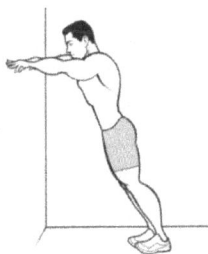

Be sure to complete the warm-up exercises we discussed earlier prior to starting these more challenging exercises.

Then, finish your workout vigorously with cool-down exercises.
Wall Pushup

This is an excellent exercise to get started on your training because it's an exercise that is moderate in intensity and gradually helps you transition into the more demanding exercises.

To perform the exercise, put your hands on the wall, while you are standing straight. Step back in such an angle so that you are leaning towards the wall.

Remove yourself from the wall but don't take away your arms. Lean towards the wall again and repeat the process. Perform about 20 times.

Alligator Pushup

This is a distinct and more difficult variation of a traditional pushup. It increases your core strength as well as upper-body strength and builds the pectoral muscles. Here's a photo that shows the pectoral muscles.

For this exercise begin by getting into the pushup position , and place one hand slightly in front of the other to the floor.

Reduce yourself gently , and then push up. Keep both your legs straight. Reverse your hand and place your other hand in front.

Then lower yourself to the next pushup after you go. Repeat the exercise for around 20 times. This video will show you how to do this exercise.

Straight Bar Dips

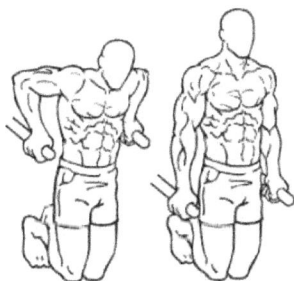

If you find it easy to perform the dips exercises in earlier chapters, switch to this one. This is a tougher version than the one before and will strengthen the chest muscles. For the exercise, sit between two bars that are straight.

Set both hands onto the bar and lower yourself as you do this, lean over the bar, trying to keep your equilibrium. This will make your abdominal muscles work more and helps strengthen your shoulders.

Check that your shoulders don't sag while you are lowering your back. Also , make sure that your elbows point directly in front of you.

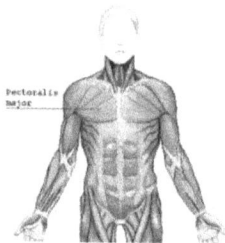

Make sure you go to the bottom while doing the dip. The goal is to have your chest reach the bar, and to maintain an angle of 90 degrees to the elbows' outsides as the weight is dropped.

Perform about 10 repetitions in this workout. Once you are proficient at it, increase the number of repetitions until 15 and then 20.

Lawn Extensions for Mowers

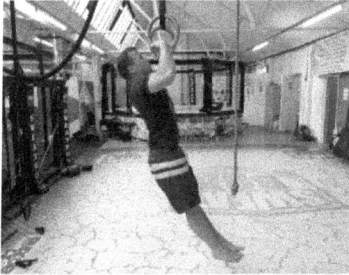

This intermediate to advanced exercise is designed to strengthen your biceps, triceps, and back. You will require gymnast rings for this workout. Make sure they are 12-18 inches off the ground. Here's how you can do the exercise:

Place your feet on your back and flat, just under your gymnast rings. Keep the ring in place, making sure your grip is solid.

With all your strength and all your strength, attempt to lift yourself from the ground, and slowly lower yourself. Start

with 10 repetitions at the beginning, and
then increase up to 20, 30, or even 30
reps.

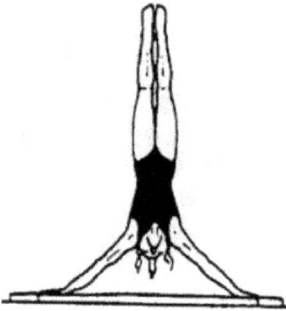

Dragon Walk

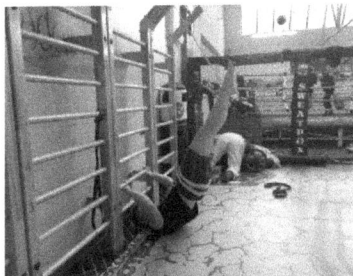

This exercise is extremely strenuous and requires you to move toward the ground, while keeping the pushups in place similar to a komodo dragon. It is a challenging practice and should be performed after you get grasp of pushups with alligators. To perform it:

Make sure you are in that pushup pose. Set one hand in front over the other. Then, raise yourself before lowering yourself back down. While you drop yourself down, shift your body in a forward direction. Move your other hand forward and then move your body towards the front.

Start with 5 minutes initially before gradually increasing this until 10 minutes.

Here's a short video that will show you how to complete the exercise properly.

Pike Pushup

This is a great exercise that will help build the strength of your upper body. When you've mastered this workout, you'll be able to do handstands. Here's how to perform the exercise:

In the A-frame position, get yourself into the posture. Your legs should be straight and wide with your arms resting on the floor with your head tucked between them.

Lower your head slowly towards the floor as the elbows are bent. Be sure to look straight through your legs. Your eyes should not be directed toward the ground. Then, push yourself up.

Perform about 20 repetitions.

Watch this video to gain a better understanding of the exercise.

Muscle-ups using Rings

This is an amazing exercise that will strengthen your body , especially your arms. Here's how to do it.

Place yourself just behind the rings. Set the rings up in such a way that they are at least an inch apart.

Take the rings by your thumbs and forefingers. Then grasp the rings in such a way where your hands are elevated. Your fingers must point downwards. Keep your elbows in close proximity to your body.

You can now you can pull yourself up and attempt to climb up as high as you can. Next, move downwards going into a dip. As you do this and then gently pull your elbows back in a manner that rotates them.

Start with 10 repetitions at the beginning, and gradually increase it to 15.

Handstands

Handstands are excellent for building your core strength as well as increasing the endurance and power of your body. They exercise your entire body , specifically the arms and hands. As your arms and hands become stronger the grip strength and strength increases; this can help you do all of the calisthenics workouts efficiently.

If you've never attempted handstands before, it's best to practice it with the assistance of a companion. Here's how to perform the handstand:

Make sure that you are standing straight and your feet are securely placed to the earth. Make sure your torso, head, feet and knees are straight and aligned. Maintain your arms by your sides.

Whichever leg you are dominant left or right kick it, then move it ahead until you are able to perform the lunge. The dominant leg must be bent while the other leg should be straight. You should now tilt your entire body forwards , allowing it to fall over the bent leg in such an order that your body is similar to the shape of an open-ended seesaw.

Keep both arms straight while gently moving your head toward the ground. Get a partner to assist you to the position of a handstand. Be careful not to put your hands on the floor because it could cause you to fall forward.

Make sure that both arms are straight as your hands touch the ground . Then, gently lift your legs and torso towards the ceiling. Make sure your legs are in line to avoid falling into the side. Request your friend to let you go once you're sure that you are able to maintain the position on your own.

Hold the position for one minute at the beginning, with help from outside. When you are able to do a handstand by yourself for a minute, gradually increase the time until you are able to do this for 10 minutes.

Dragon Flags

It's both a long and enjoyable exercise perform. This exercise strengthens your arms, abs and legs and builds your arm, calf and ab muscles. Here's the best way to perform the exercise:

Place your feet on the floor straight. Grab any low lying sturdy object or low bar. Be sure your hands are up above your head.

Then, lift both feet so that the entire weight of your body is on your shoulders while your toes are pointed towards the sky. You may want to secure your feet using the help of a band before you begin.

Then slowly lower your feet toward the floor. Make sure that you remain with your body as level as possible. If you're doing it right your body will appear like a hinge , and your abs will hold your whole body in place as you lower your body towards the floor.

Do 10 repetitions at the beginning. If you feel it is too difficult try 5 repetitions.

Plyometric Body Row

Also known by the name of Australian Pullups, this type of exercise is an awesome variation on the traditional pull-up and will strengthen your shoulders and arms, to perform tougher exercises with ease. You'll require a sturdy bar that is low for this workout. The bar should be in the middle of your hip prior to starting the exercise. Here's how you can perform the exercise

Lay flat onto your stomach. Hold the bar in your hands.

Concentrate on the upwards and forcefully strive to raise yourself. While doing that you pull your shoulders backwards. Make sure to pull yourself upwards fast so that you can release the bar at the bottom and grasp it just before you get to the lowest point.

Do 10 repetitions If it's easy for you or if you find it difficult try 5 reps.

Here's a video that the explanation of the exercise.

Handstand Pushups

Once you've gotten into the routine of pike pushups your strength will improve dramatically and you'll be able to perform pushups with hands. Here's how to do pushups:

Face a wall and stand. Your feet should be raised in such a way that you're standing hand-to-hand against the wall.

Then, squeeze your abs, glutes, and thigh muscles on both legs. Slowly lower yourself to the floor as much as you are able to.

Do the push-ups and repeat this process. Perform 10 repetitions if it is possible.

Take a look at this video for instructions on how to do this exercise.

Flag Pole

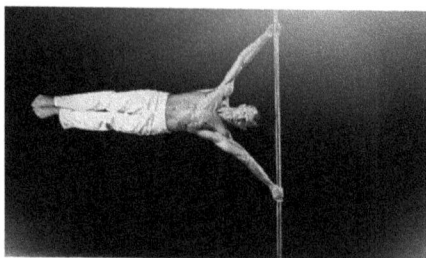

This is an extremely tough exercise but it boosts the strength, stamina and endurance in a multitude of ways. Although it's difficult to master, If you regularly do pull-ups and handstand push-ups often and regularly, you'll be able complete this exercise. Here's how to perform this exercise:

Place yourself next to a vertical pole that has been planted to the floor. It is best to choose an inch thick pole because it is much easier to grasp and hold on to.

Secure the pole using both hands and ensure that both arms are straight.

Once you feel that your grip is firm enough then use your upper arm to pull yourself slowly up , while your lower arm presses against the pole to support your body.

Continue to pull your body upwards until you're perpendicular to the pole, and then you can make an eagle.

It's recommended to start with the exercises described at the start of the chapter. Then, gradually progress to more advanced exercises. You can mix a few exercises to create your own routine according to the muscles you would like to develop. It is important to conclude your workout with cooling down exercises.

Chapter 19: How to Create A Mindset That Will Find Calisthenics

The concept of the specificity principle is a fancy way of saying you'll get better in the specific things you practice. In the event that you wish to progress in a specific exercise, you need to do it with a specific procedure.

The muscle-up could be an amazing illustration of. There are lots of athletes who do not believe in the muscle-up at the beginning. I certainly did! However, no matter how strong you're or the number of pull-ups you're able to accomplish, the muscle-up simply a distinct move that needs to be repeated until it gets more fluid.

It's similar to how one could be a fantastic musician, however if they wish to learn how to play the cello, they must still practice their cello!

So many people give excuses for why they are unable to find healthful and sometimes even remain consistent with their exercise regimen. You may have heard phrases like as,"I really don't have time," or even"that the gym isn't as good," or even"my kids are taking up the majority of my time " There are many explanations for this. In reality, everyone is able to accomplish. The issue is that the vast majority of people do not wish to. They are searching for a magic potion for a healthier lifestyle. Folks, let me say that there are no pills.

To be fit, you need to be healthy. Modifying the way that you think about the fitness is an important part of the overall solution. It's a mental shift.

How you think about fitness starts with the attitude you have towards it. It could originate from your young, the ones you are the least and so on. The people who have been lifelong athletes are often able to maintain this mentality. Fitness is a one of the main goals of everyday life. People of all ages particularly in our modern times tend to fall into the category of couch potato. Most people aren't even engaged with their bodies.

To create a mentality to Fitness Center, you have do it. The reason is the increasing popularity of practices. In the present, you may be thinking,"If I'm not going to have the mindset to be fit is that you are saying I must be healthy?" It's a little. The majority of athletes are naturally drawn to exercise because they've previously done this for the majority times throughout their lives. It's a way of life for them.

What I'm telling you to do is always to start taking on any kind of action based on a specific goal and plan. Start small and gradually take it up. I'll provide you with some strategies that will allow you to achieve this mindset quicker.

A great Way that has helped many Is through visualization. Imagine you're an athlete performing the kind of exercises they engage in. Be sure to keep this in the future in your the mind. What you want to achieve is to achieve this goal. These are the reasons why working by setting a goal, it is crucial. Aiming for a goal is likely to motivate you to exercise.

Any physical act you perform for a cause can assist in the pursuit of the goal to get there. A constant and increasing amount of challenges will keep you focused. Working out with athletes can help in forming this mentality. The most common expression is that we are the average of the five people we are correlated with the highest. In the event you are able to connect with physically fit people, you're likely to be like them. You must be able to upon fitness-focused people in your local community as well as on social media websites like Facebook.

One tool that can keep your Track is a diary. Find one and begin using it. What you want to do be able to keep an eye on your daily actions. Record everything you've accomplished regarding physical exercise and also the foods you ate to nourish and fuel your system to operate. The simple method of writing down these details helps to establish in your subconscious mind that you're fit. If you've got some obstacles that you have just conquered and met the goal, write it down, too. It's a reflection of what you've accomplished within your mental.

BTW every activity that puts you in a difficult position is a good thing. It is not necessary to get to the gym to get a great workout. If you have a fitness mindset that is a workout mindset, you'll realize that anything is your own personal gym. I recently made use of all the equipment I could find in a hotel room to work out. For my own spine , I only dragged myself up to the top edge of the desk. I let my body hang below and did the human body's weight in pops. I was able to do squats with human body weight and push-ups. I have no reason that I can give for the reasons why I was unable to workout. It was just me who did this. It was my mindset that led me to find out what I could do.

A lot of us who talk about the subject of health and wellness speak about"getting fit again" What they aren't aware of is that often these words can be contrary to the aim of actually becoming fit. It's commonplace to hear people complaining about being in poor shape and saying"that I'm looking to improve my fitness and shed fat", and"that I wish to lose weight and be fit". But what's not often said in conjunction with these expressions is the idea of"and remain the same"and stay this".

While staying fit may be their goal however, their mind is only focused on the short-term aim of becoming fit. This mindset is a common cause of many people who are susceptible to the latest diet regimens and fitness gimmicks that are available on the market. Therefore, we're committed to becoming fit and healthy in the shortest period of time . We will take on any challenge, no matter how ridiculous or difficult it might be to use... or hazardous or unhealthy!

Making changes to our"Quickfix" Mindset to a lasting success mindset and lifestyle changes can help us to follow the right and sustainable way. You could soon find yourself less attracted to late night television advertisements and more focused on doing the right thing at the appropriate times. Aren't a lengthy, long-lasting, happy life what we really want?

Making the ideal environment that allows the body to eliminate fat quickly is crucial to your goal and takes lots of work. It's much easier to remain in healthy in your 30's and your 20's than when you're in your 60's and 50's... as you'll age, and get fitter which is impressive! It's rare to meet people who have maintained their mentality and followed an regimen of exercise and nutrition that has helped them stay healthier.

If you truly want to transform how you feel about Human body and well-being forever, you have to ensure that it's a habit. It should be engrained by the things you experience and the way you think. There is no need to be thinking about eating foods that are healthy but it's likely to be something you do because you love it! Studies have shown that these habits could be established in a matter of a month and in some cases, faster. You don't have to give your life's dreams a chance and you do not have to adhere to the latest diet trend.

Losing weight isn't as difficult as many people make to make it appear. Personally, I think that the media can make losing weight appear to be more difficult than it really is. and I believe this is precisely why it's actually a multi-billion dollar year market.

The Truth is That the old-fashioned way of eating and exercising will allow you to shed weight. but the mentality that the media has shaped us believe with us that standard methods aren't working anymore.

Below are a couple of suggestions that will provide you with the right attitude to slim down:

1.) Choose something that is effective...

The decision to purchase an item or method, that Works is one of the key components. With all the frauds out there, deciding on the best product could be difficult. Ensure that you purchase from a reputable source or don't spend too much dollars on the item in case it appears to be too good to be true.

2.) remain ...

This must be the most crucial aspect. You have a decent product, all you need to do is remain with this. An additional week's study has been released by a major health website that sells supplements , so when they asked consumers if try the product once they got it, an amazing 50% did not say no!

We've become pretty inactive, I think and that only proves it. The best thing you can do is remain the same. Some of the things that could help you stick to your goal could include putting up a picture of yourself a few years ago, as if you're a lot more attractive than the one on your refrigerator.

If you ever need to go out for a bite you'll be gazing back at the mirror of your former self.

Whatever you choose to do, or choose not, the most important thing is to always be aware and far from all of the Scams that are available.

Pushing exercises and pulling exercises

It is essential to be aware of the drawing exercises you're performing in contrast to the number of challenging exercises you're performing specifically for your body. A few instances of pulling exercises for the torso are pull-ups lap pull-downs, dumbbell rows and so on.. There are many instances of hammering exercises on the torso comprise dumbbell presses, pushups, bench presses and so on.. The general rule is that yanking exercises could be beneficial to your Biceps, while exercises that shove may be a good way to work your waist. You may not realize that you're pulling a lot and your biceps become painful. It's important to remain alert and aware that you're not overworking your muscles. Pulling and pushing are often two different things. It is important to be aware of the particulars when you are making configurations to get the most benefit.

Super collection is a method to combine two exercises so that you get the most out of your endurance and time. However, if you do two push-up exercises and then you'll begin to strain your shoulders or your triceps. There are exceptions to this principle. But, you shouldn't try to perform repetitive movements with no understanding of what you may be doing. For example, if you find that you do only 1 or 2 repetitions of bench presses, it would be ineffective to do 1 or 2 repetitions of the heavy dumbbell seat presses. Your shoulders and waist could be injured while performing 2-4 repetitions of bench presses that are heavy. Although it seems trivial, it's important to fully be aware of the concept of pushing and pulling. How can that understanding aid me in creating my own amazing collection or mix of specific moves?

As you are aware of the thought of Pulling and Pushing and pulling, you can test out exactly what exercises be performed in great collection. Pullups and push-ups are great for working out. This is a very driving type of exercise. Another alternative is drawing type of exercise. Press yards and bench back are amazing super workouts that can be set. It is not necessary to wear your elbows back and shoulders, shoulders or knees. However, you're sure to find a workout combination that will maximize your effort and result. Dum-bell curls as well as dumb bell kick-backs are a combination of exercises. One of them targets your shoulder (yanking) and the other is a waist workout (pushing). This will help you save joints from pain.

Thus, it's crucial to remember that pushing pulling exercises and push-ups. There are some slight variations to this principle. It is a common that pros deliberately place various exercises. It is important to stay up to date, regardless of whether the exercise may be a pushing or pulling exercise.

The exercise of the confront is a variation of a row, utilizing the arms extended inwards throughout the execution of the exercise, so that the body's deltoid trunk gets a great deal of tension, while the upper back muscles of the flip are less engaged. To complete the exercise, you must stand within an arm's reach within the cable channel using the cable pulley that is corrected to be at the head level that is fitted with an attachment for rope. When you are standing up, place your hands on the rope handles and then draw your hands towards both sides of their heads. The arms on top should remain in a high position and be smelly and external throughout the duration of the workout. When you have a higher level of immunity, that posture could need to be altered to give greater stability and balance, such as placing one foot a few feet in front of the another.

A facial tug resembles the back deltoid, and the bent side raise, in which every exercise successfully relaxing your back shoulders mind. The isolation of this back deltoid may be beneficial during the shoulder workout in conjunction with traditional exercises for the shoulder that place only a small amount of direct stress to your back shoulder. There are a myriad of shoulder pressing exercises are excellent for stimulating the both sides of the head but they do not put much stress on your back delt(oid) head. Trainers may want to include a back shoulder workout for greater balance in the workout. Because most torso workouts include front shoulder exercises, many spinal exercises stress the back of the shoulder. Hence, it's worth noting that this muscles are subject to a significant tension during back exercises.

If there aren't any flexible cable available this procedure can be carried out using the seated cable row regardless of the fact that the immunity is likely to be from the less reputable source. If you have free weights are best seeking the back row.

You'll have the ability to create the whole body you've always wanted should you start with these best exercise routines for fat loss for both men and women. Many men invest a lot on time and money in the fitness center for days at a time, only to get very little in the kind of outcomes. You could exercise daily all night at the same time, but you will never see any significant changes if you're performing the wrong types of exercises for fat loss for both males and females.

There's an abundance of exercises to reduce fat for men to choose from. But, certain exercises can result in burning more fat quicker than other exercises. This guide will focus on the most efficient five fat-burning exercises specifically designed for both males and females to aid men in burning off more fat and build strong and healthy muscles quickly.

These exercises could also help to increase your metabolism, which can help in shedding the extra weight that can be difficult to get rid with a regular diet and exercises. What is the purpose of those high five muscle-building fat-burning exercises for both males and females?

Before we go into the details, it's Crucial to be aware of how your exercise program will fail you each time when you're not performing the correct exercises that will be successful. Don't waste your time or precious money on exercise regimens or diet plans that don't work, incorporate these effective routines beginning now to begin seeing the results.

The most essential thing you will ever learn that can help you grow into healthier and healthy is to enhance your routine on a daily basis in order to avoid getting stuck in a plateau.

Today we can talk about the most effective five-pound burning exercises for both males and females. There's one aspect you should keep in mind prior to starting your new fat loss routine for both men regularly. The exercises that are described here are more focused on the movements which need to be performed instead of a set exercise routines. For instance it is possible to do numerous exercises employing the movements that we're going to discuss that will enable the user to perform an impressive workout with a variety of kinds of exercises to help you to avoid the plateaus in your workout.

Change and numbers are the most important part of this workout program that can allow you to attain real success.

Here's the final list of the top five exercises to reduce fat in both males and females:

SQUAT MOVEMENTS

The very first thing we'll discuss in this high five fat-reducing exercises for men and women could include the use of a barbell or barbell that is integrated into the squat or the use of an old elevator or kettle-bell, barbell swing or some other similar motion that's going to give exactly the same result.

Kettlebells have been a widely used tool during Fat Burning exercise as it promotes body movement throughout the entire human body through the hips, torso and the body's centre. The body is being re-programmed throughout this particular exercise.

Squatting in this manner will allow you to reduce a significant amount of calories because it involves lots of physical and mechanical work that must be completed by the human body. This is the first step on the list of the top five exercises that reduce fat in both men and women. Always begin your fitness program with the barbell for effective exercises to burn fat both genders.

It's crucial to keep in mind that movements that are thought of as the most"squat kind" are also split-squats and exercises, however they can be used in conjunction with the single-leg exercise guidelines given below. Sometimes, the distinction between the two types could blur slightly, as they are beneficial for a variety different purposes. This is the best time to look at the forthcoming exercises for men that burn fat in our list.

Conclusion

In the present technology has transformed your life into something that is easier than it was a couple of decades ago. The technology has transformed the majority of household chores much easier and straightforward.

However the culture of computer work that is based on computers, requires users to be at your desk for about nine hours a day. This, along with poor eating habits and your consumption of harmful refined foods and pre-cooked meals that have caused a lack of appetite to be among the most significant causes of loss generally and also leads to be a part of other recurring illnesses like diabetes mellitus and osteoarthritis (erosion of joint cartilage as well as the associated bones) hypertension, bronchial asthma heart ailments and malignancies. In this state of affairs, staying in good shape with a slim, healthy and trim body is an extremely important factors in everyone's calendar.

Not just to look better, but also to live in a fit and healthy way. Being fit is not necessarily about becoming involved in a fitness club and working out with equipment or lifting heavy weights for a long time. It is possible to do it in a clean and simple method using calisthenics. However, make sure to do the exercises consistently without interruption for a single day. You can achieve a slim, muscular appearance with a slim, flat stomach and toned legs in a brief amount of time.